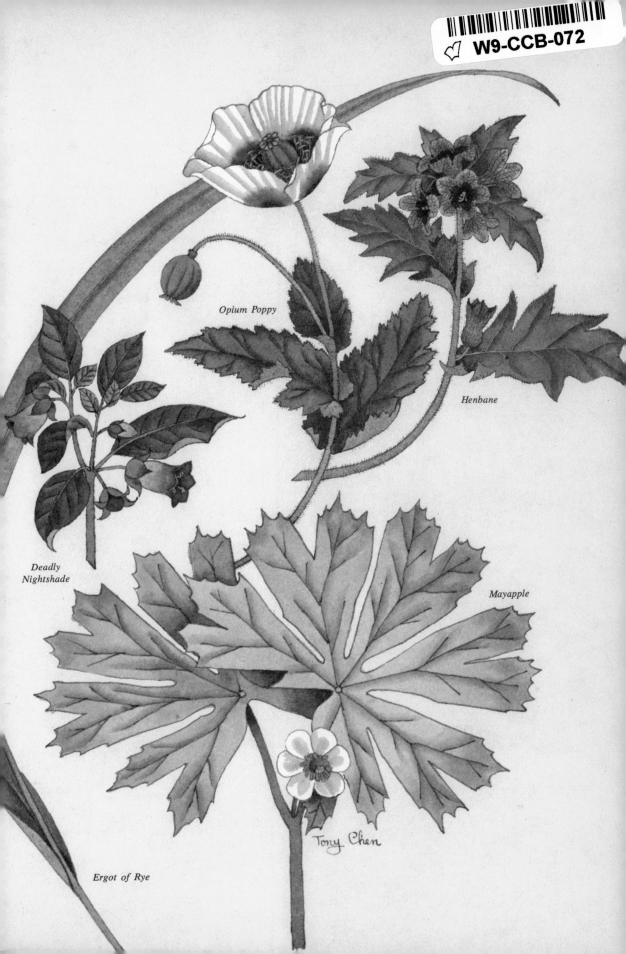

Opium Poppy

Henbane

Deadly
Nightshade

Mayapple

Tony Chen

Ergot of Rye

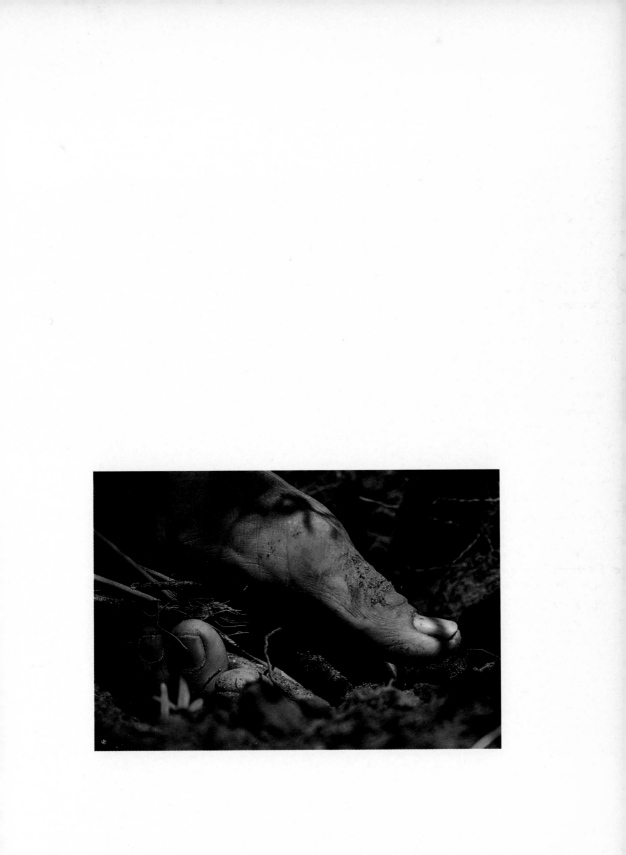

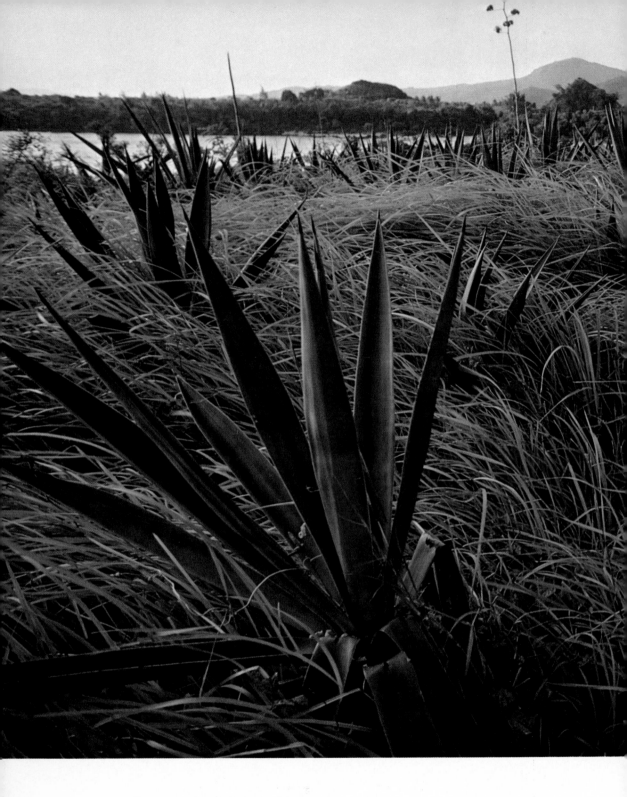

By Lonnelle Aikman
Photographs by Nathan Benn and Ira Block
Prepared by the Special Publications Division
National Geographic Society, Washington, D. C.

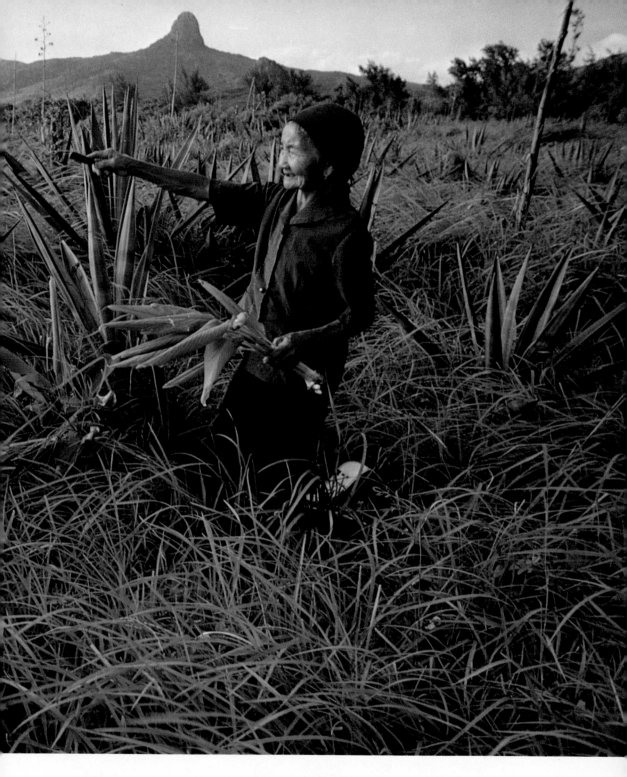

Nature's Healing Arts
From Folk Medicine to Modern Drugs

NATURE'S HEALING ARTS: FROM FOLK MEDICINE TO MODERN DRUGS

By LONNELLE AIKMAN
Photographs by NATHAN BENN *and* IRA BLOCK
Paintings by TONY CHEN

Published by
THE NATIONAL GEOGRAPHIC SOCIETY
ROBERT E. DOYLE, *President*
MELVIN M. PAYNE, *Chairman of the Board*
GILBERT M. GROSVENOR, *Editor*
MELVILLE BELL GROSVENOR, *Editor Emeritus*

Prepared by
THE SPECIAL PUBLICATIONS DIVISION
ROBERT L. BREEDEN, *Editor*
DONALD J. CRUMP, *Associate Editor*
PHILIP B. SILCOTT, *Senior Editor*
WILLIAM R. GRAY, *Managing Editor*
MARJORIE W. CLINE, *Senior Researcher;*
  BONNIE S. LAWRENCE, *Researcher*

Illustrations and Design
THOMAS B. POWELL III, *Picture Editor*
JODY BOLT, *Art Director*
SUEZ B. KEHL, *Assistant Art Director*
CHRISTINE K. ECKSTROM, DAVID R. FINDLEY,
  H. ROBERT MORRISON, JENNIFER C. URQUHART,
  EDWARD O. WELLES, JR., *Picture Legends*

Production and Printing
ROBERT W. MESSER, *Production Manager*
GEORGE V. WHITE, *Assistant Production
  Manager*
RAJA D. MURSHED, JUNE L. GRAHAM,
  CHRISTINE A. ROBERTS, *Production Assistants*
JOHN R. METCALFE, *Engraving and Printing*
DEBRA A. ANTONINI, JANE H. BUXTON,
  SUZANNE J. JACOBSON, AMY E. METCALFE,
  CLEO PETROFF, DAVID V. SHOWERS,
  KATHERYN M. SLOCUM, SUZANNE VENINO,
  MARILYN L. WILBUR, *Staff Assistants*
MARTHA K. HIGHTOWER, *Index*

*Overleaf: Chinese herbalist in Taiwan picks
yellow ginger in a field spiked with agave plants. A
familiar spice, ginger also soothes stomach
disorders. Page 1: Navajo medicine man in
Arizona eases out an* oshá *root, used to combat
the common cold. Endsheets: Classics of
medicine — plants from around the world yield
remedies for illnesses ranging from headaches to
cancer. Bookbinding: An herb enthusiast gathers
mullein in the mountains of southern Virginia.*

OVERLEAF AND PAGE 1: NATHAN BENN; ENDSHEETS: TONY CHEN;
BOOKBINDING: JODY BOLT FROM A PHOTOGRAPH BY IRA BLOCK

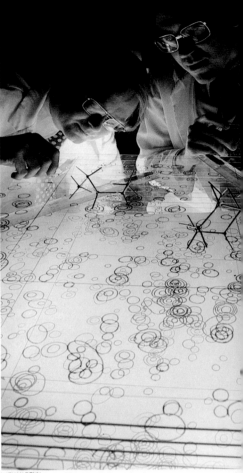

NATHAN BENN

*Scientists at Eli Lilly and Company,
a pharmaceutical firm based in
Indianapolis, plot the molecular
structure of an antibiotic.
Medicinal plants — nature's gift
to man — provide chemical
blueprints for synthetic drugs.*

Foreword

A CRISP, SALT-TINGED BREEZE nudged our sloop along the rocky coast of Rhode Island. I had cruised here many times to poke among the islands and coves in search of marine life for my chemical and pharmacological studies. As always, I reflected on the wealth of beneficial substances given to mankind by nature. I was sailing on water rich with life, and past land abundant with wild plants that have already provided important medicines; I wondered at the number of species which have not yet been examined for their potential as drugs that heal.

I first became interested in medicinal plants through my late father, Heber Youngken, Sr., who was known as the dean of American pharmacognosists—those scientists who derive drugs from natural sources. As a boy, I accompanied him on many field trips. He would entertain me with stories of the medical and folklore uses of a particular flower, leaf, fruit, root, or seed. Later, studying under Dr. Merritt Fernald of Harvard, I visited Cape Cod, and learned how Indians there had cured their ills with dune grass, dusty miller, and bog weeds. Such days would end with Dr. Fernald's scalloped oyster casserole made with wild herbs.

As a scientist, I have devoted my career to drug plants. My colleagues and I, trying to understand and duplicate the workings of natural drugs, have had some successes, but many failures. As with Humpty Dumpty, it is often impossible to put the pieces together again to reproduce the action of nature in curing a disease. It is also difficult to match the natural functions of plants known for centuries to people who have practiced folk medicine: the heart-saving effect of digitalis in the foxglove plant; the invigorating quality of ginseng; the expectorant action of wild-cherry bark.

Such natural wonders interest not just scientists. In growing numbers, people across the nation—in the city as well as the country—are looking back to traditional healing plants as sources of drugs. In this book, author Lonnelle Aikman surveys the world of medicinal plants—from folklore uses of herbal remedies to scientific attempts to regulate disease with botanical drugs. In so doing, she brings to life not only the plants, but also the people who use them in the home and in the laboratory.

There are real dangers in self-medication with herbal remedies, however. The old adage that goes, "if a small dose works, a bigger dose works better," does not necessarily hold. For many plants can cause unpleasant side effects, and some are deadly poisonous. It is always important to know what you are using and what its results are; careless dosing can lead to dangerous complications.

Still, searching for medications from nature is a never-ending challenge. Each time I moor my sloop in a cove and begin to look for land and sea organisms, I wonder which species from nature's storehouse will be the next cure for a disease that has plagued mankind for centuries.

HEBER W. YOUNGKEN, JR., PH.D.

Professor of Pharmacognosy, University of Rhode Island

Contents

*Arkansas native Billy Joe Tatum
samples wild honey taken from
a bee tree. Used for millennia, this
vitamin-rich food forms a basic
ingredient of many folk remedies.*

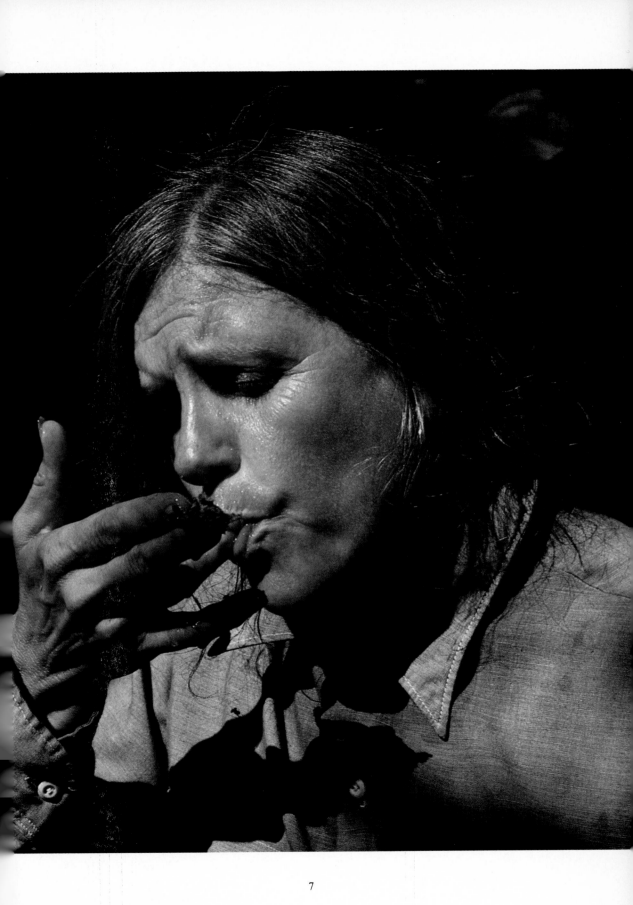

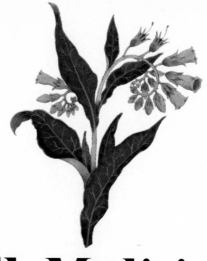

Folk Medicine:
An Enduring Art

THE TEMPERATURE had climbed to a stifling 90 degrees in the shade when I parked along a narrow country road deep in the Ozarks of Missouri. Fanning myself with a map, I walked into the spacious yard of the person I had come to visit.

She was sitting under a big Japanese umbrella, despite the thick woods around her and the great branches arching overhead. Dressed in an ample, flowing muumuu, her gray hair clipped short, her legs propped up on a footstool, she looked like an amiable Buddha surrounded by followers—in this case, a small group of friends. A beige-colored gibbon, chattering and swinging from branch to branch in a nearby tree, added to the exotic atmosphere.

The scene was not exactly what I had pictured when I decided to visit Monty Pope to learn about folk medicine in the Ozarks. Nor is Monty any stereotype of a simple country woman. A onetime ballet teacher and the author of a small book of sensitive poems about nature, she is described by her friends as a "lady with a heart as big as she is."

Yet behind the wildly improbable stage setting in which I found her, Monty Pope, I quickly discovered, is an *(Continued on page 16)*

Gathering wild herbs near her Arkansas home, Billy Joe Tatum picks horsemint for a medicinal tea. Many scientists, physicians—and enthusiasts like Billy Joe—rely on nature's pharmacy for plants that heal.

COMFREY (ABOVE)

NICK KELSH

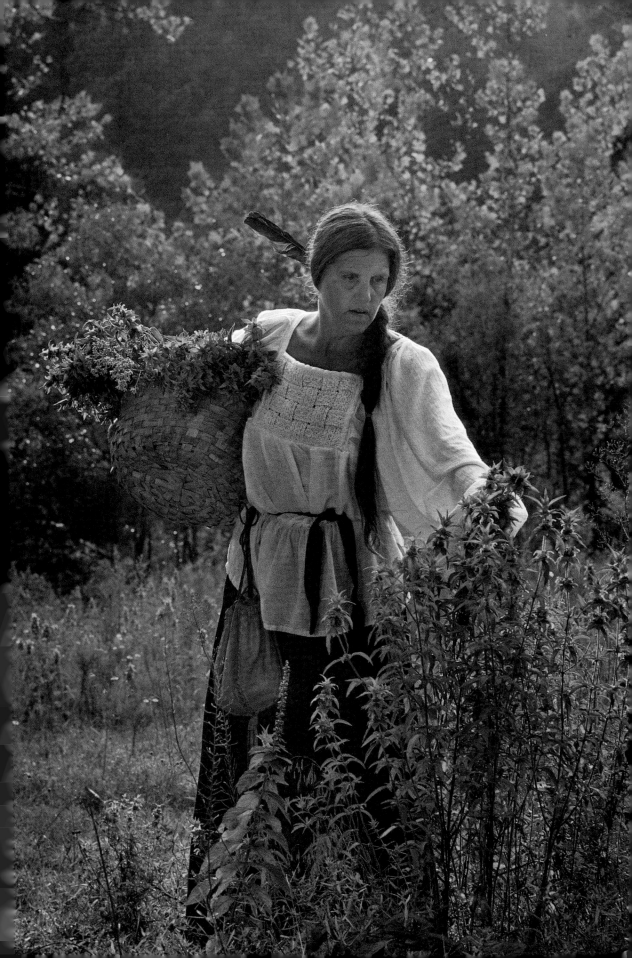

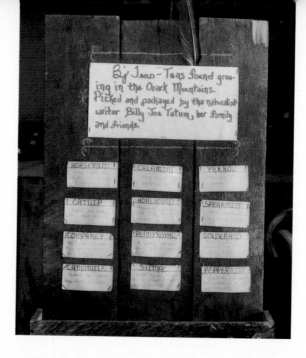

Beneath a jagged bluff, Billy Joe Tatum wades Little Piney Creek in search of wild mint and horsetail reeds for soothing teas. "Old-time remedies taste good!" she says, describing the fragrant herb teas (above) that her family sells at a craft shop. Her husband, Dr. Harold Tatum, joins a growing number of physicians who occasionally prescribe herbal medicines. Outside his clinic in Melbourne, Arkansas, he treats two poison ivy sufferers with Aloe vera (below). Breaking the fleshy leaf, he squeezes the clear liquid onto his patients' rashes to relieve itching.

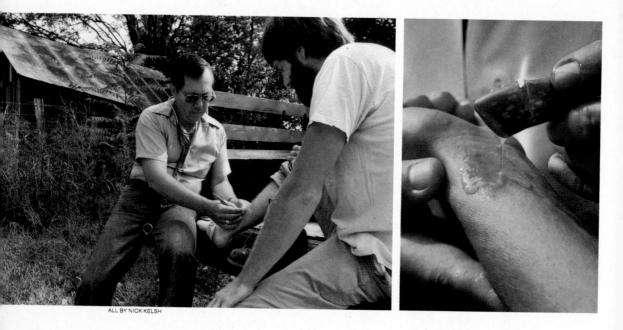

ALL BY NICK KELSH

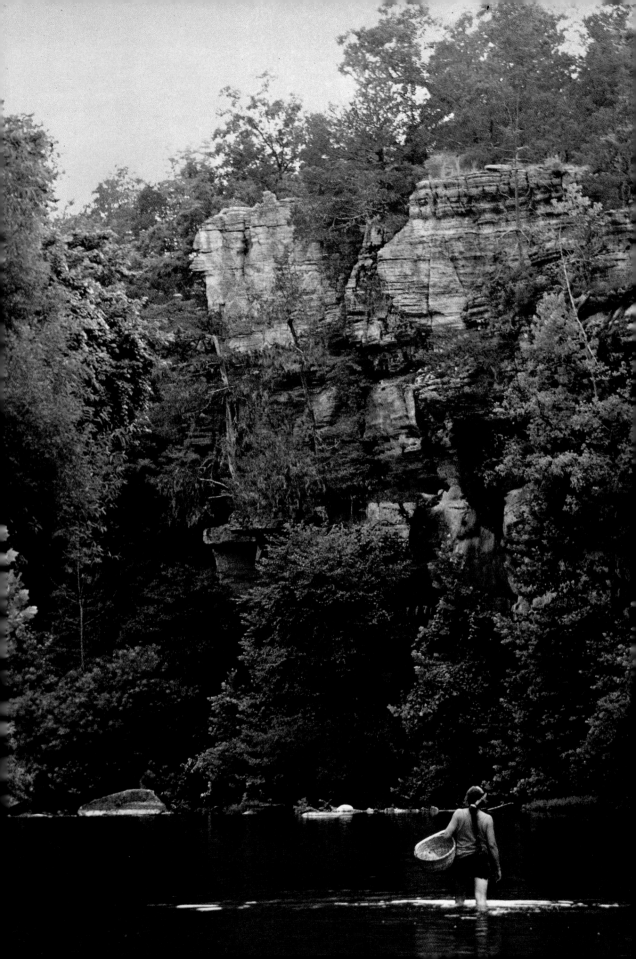

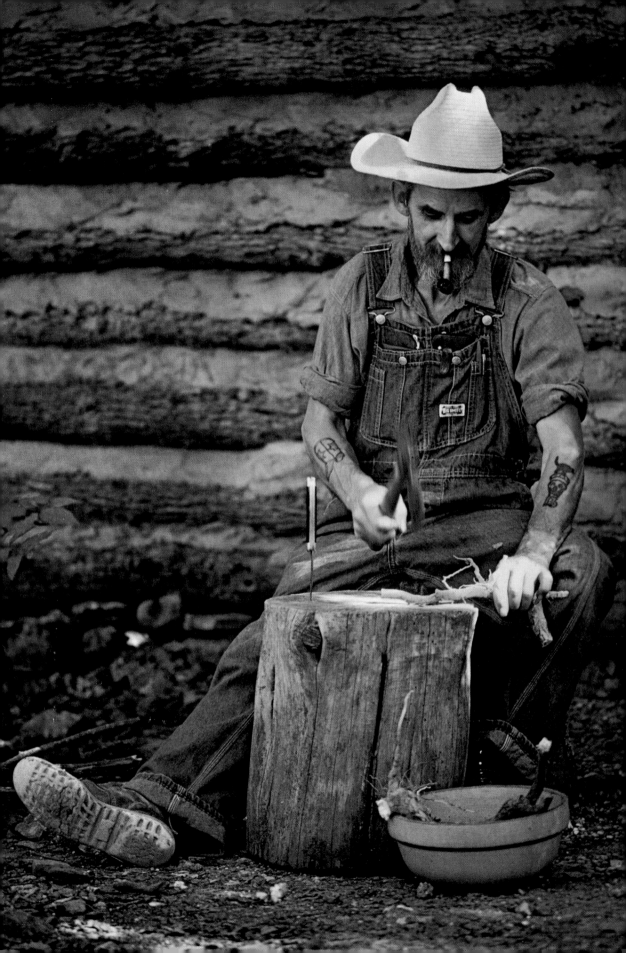

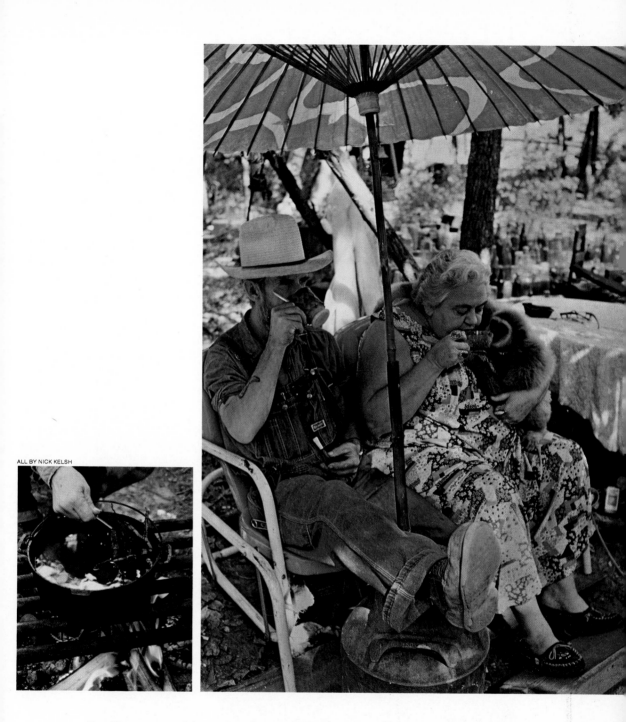

Cradling a pet gibbon, Ozark native Monty Pope shares sassafras tea with friend Billy Hebner on her farm near Branson, Missouri. In the hilly woodlands around her home, she collects wild plants for both food and medicine. "Every day here we tap the source of what pharmacists use in their capsules and pills," she says. At left, Billy chops fresh sassafras root, then boils it in spring water (above) to extract its sweet flavors.

13

Country medicines endure in the Ozarks: At her home in Walnut Shade, Missouri, Ella Dunn sips hot spicebush tea as her companion, Ruth Branstetter, reads a book. Mrs. Dunn enjoys the restorative as a coffee substitute, adding, "If you make it strong, it will run a fever down." Herb fancier Mainard Rasnick (bottom) swallows a dose of his homemade pokeroot tonic, a fiery medicine made with 100-proof whiskey that he takes for arthritis. Relaxing on the porch of his Arkansas home, Waco Johnson teaches his grandson to smoke mullein—a popular decongestant.

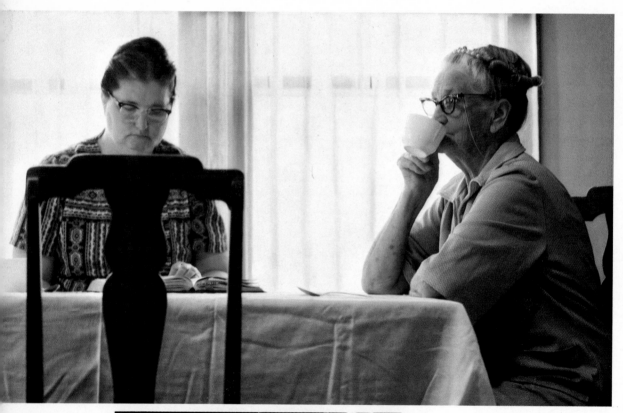

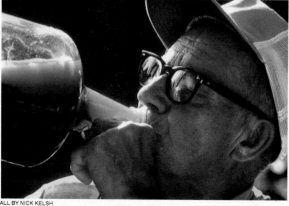

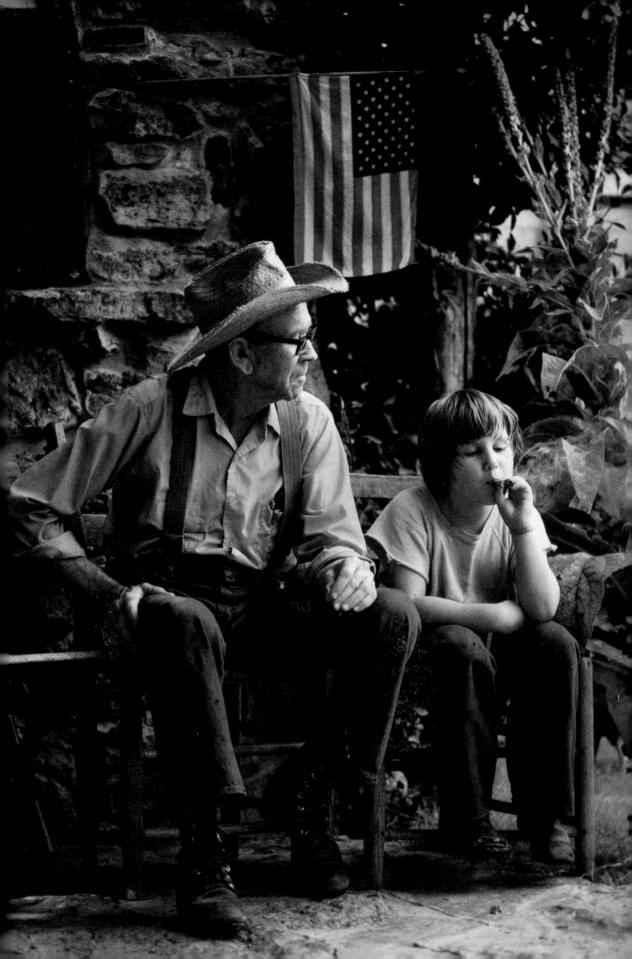

authentic Ozarkian, rooted in the soil in the best folk tradition. "My great-grandfather was one of the earliest homesteaders around here," she said. "This land, 160 acres of it, has been in my family for a hundred years. Land grabbers keep trying to get me to sell it, but I wouldn't take a million dollars for it. Living here makes me happy, and the land gives me a lot.

"I don't have to go farther than my yard for beneficial herbs," said Monty as we walked along winding, tree-shaded paths on her property. "If I can beat the possums to them, I take persimmons and blackberries when they are just ripe; they're so good for you then with all their vitamins and minerals.

"I eat wild violet blossoms for their high vitamin C content, and for greens there's wild lettuce, lamb's-quarters, dandelions, dock, purslane, and cattails. Either tossed in a salad or sautéed, they're succulent and healthful. I also like that greenbrier over there," she said, pointing to a bright green meandering vine. "In spring you can break off its young shoots like asparagus and eat them raw. They're full of minerals, and they clean your teeth and leave your mouth feeling astringent.

"I'm always very careful about the plants I use, but once I made a mistake by brewing a tea with the big leaves of mullein and keeping it around till it got too strong. I'd been having trouble sleeping, so I took the mullein as a sedative. I slept that night, but I had wild, unsettling nightmares. Next morning I threw out the rest of that tea.

"Actually," Monty continued with pride, "I've seldom been sick since I moved back here from the city. I am beginning to feel the pangs of arthritis, however, and I plan to start a research campaign to find wild plants that might control or maybe cure it. Meantime, my favorite medicinal drink is still a tea made with sassafras root. I call it my wonder drink because it's a muscle toner, an astringent, and good for your skin. I drank a lot of it with sugar and cream when I was a teenager, and I never had any skin problems."

Back at the Japanese umbrella after our walk in the woods, Monty served a special tea. Brewed in an iron pot over a flaming campfire, it contained fresh spring water, pennyroyal, yarrow, hound's-tongue, wild peppermint, and honey.

It tasted sweet and mild, and each of the ingredients goes into everyday prescriptions of Ozark herbalists: pennyroyal for anything from insect bites to convulsions; yarrow for colds and fevers; hound's-tongue and wild peppermint for headaches or gastric disorders.

Such use of natural products—leaves, barks, roots, blossoms, and other parts of herbs and trees—is almost as old as mankind. In fact, the botanical kingdom was by far the main source of all drugs until synthetics came of age during the present century.

Even today, more than 40 percent of all prescription drugs sold each year in the United States are made up, at least partly, of natural products. Moreover, this figure may well be increased as a result of new sources of plant drugs and improved methods of extracting and processing, according to Dr. Norman R. Farnsworth, professor of pharmacognosy at the University of Illinois, and past president of the American Society of Pharmacognosy. He regards the prospect as "the sleeping giant of drug development in the U.S.A."

Other specialists in pharmacognosy — the science that deals specifically with natural raw materials used in drug compounds — agree with Dr. Farnsworth's prediction. A contributing factor, they point out, is the worldwide movement to return to nature's handouts.

Part of this human yearning for what is natural and old-fashioned may be attributed to a reaction against the growing pollution and mechanization of modern life, coupled with the fear that chemicals in synthetic drugs may have harmful side effects. Or maybe it's just the perennial nostalgia that charms us all.

Whatever the cause, it is easy to find evidence of the trend in the number of people undertaking organic farming, in the diverse groups studying medicinal herbs and their application, and in the enthusiasm of an increasing number of college students who are choosing to major in pharmacognosy.

Most exciting of all is the rising interest of marine biologists and other marine scientists in fishing for drugs from the sea. In this fast-expanding field, exploring divers already have discovered undersea organisms that hold useful drug compounds.

During my own research in preparing an article called "Nature's Gifts to Medicine," published in the September 1974 NATIONAL GEOGRAPHIC magazine, I had talked with leading pharmacognosists who believed that the future of medicine lies in going to both land and sea for natural products that would yield new drugs.

Now I, too, was hitting the nature trail in the Ozarks. Eventually the quest would take me, or the photographers assigned to illustrate this book, across the United States, to Central America, to the Caribbean, to Europe, Africa, and Asia. It would lead to museums and libraries exhibiting medical relics and medieval and ancient herbals, and to ultramodern laboratories equipped with instruments to analyze therapeutic substances extracted from plant, animal, and mineral products.

Along the way I would meet and make friends with many rare characters who generously shared their herbal lore and technical knowledge with me, from simple country people living deep in the woods without modern conveniences, to erudite professors whose conversation bristled with tongue-twisting terms I had to use a dictionary to understand.

In the Ozarks, one of the first of these helpful collaborators was a veteran herb enthusiast, Mainard Rasnick, who grows most of his own medicine on a large lot surrounding his modest white stucco home in Branson, Missouri — population 2,500.

17

"This wild cherry is a medical tree," he told me as we toured his living pharmacy. "I make a cough syrup from the bark. The syrup is also supposed to be a good heart tonic."

In his striped overalls and red shirt, Mr. Rasnick reminded me of a proud farmer showing off bumper crops as we passed each cluster of his precious plants—many denounced elsewhere as pests and lawn spoilers. "Here are my dandelions," he said. "I make a medicine out of the roots that's good for kidney trouble. Same with the plantain broadleaf growing over there.

"Now we're getting into my violets," he went on. "I use their leaves in a tea for a blood purifier. And I take the roots of that yellow dock for the same thing. My herb book says it's the best blood purifier in the world."

One after another, Rasnick identified his plants and explained their uses. "The roots of that poke by the big trees down there," he said, indicating a thick plant nearly ten feet tall, "I put in a medicine for arthritis. To keep it from spoiling, I fill the bottle full of 100-proof whiskey. It's too powerful for some folks even in eyedropper doses. Others around here say it takes the pain and stiffness right out of them."

I saw wild lettuce growing: "Squeeze out its white milk on a wart," said Rasnick, "and they say the wart will fall off." Slippery elm: "You take the inside of the bark and make a powder and then a drink, and it heals and soothes a sick stomach." Elder: "Every part of it is good for medicine—the flowers, the berries, the leaves, and the bark."

Invited into his house, I had a sip of homemade cough syrup much less fiery than the poke remedy he makes for arthritis. Besides its base of boiled horehound leaves, stems, and blossoms, it contained wild cherry bark and berries, anise seeds, red clover, sugar, and a touch of whiskey—and it tasted fine.

I also met Mr. Rasnick's paralyzed wife, Joyce, whom he looks after tenderly. "I make a tea for her out of the blossoms, stems, and leaves of the alfalfa you saw blooming," he said. "That's for her arthritis. She has a doctor who gives her diuretics for a weak heart. There's also a medicine for the same thing made from wild grapevine root.

"My grandpa, who was a doctor and supposed to be a pretty good heart man back in those days, used to give it to his patients. In fact, he made most of his own medicines. For the wild grapevine one, he would burn the roots into a black ash. Then he gave a spoonful in water, and it worked as good as any diuretic."

Finally, Rasnick showed me his room-size medicine chest—a shed in the back lot that was redolent with a mixture of diverse smells. Neatly labeled bottles holding all sorts of dried herbs stood on shelves along the wall. He opened some of them for me to sniff, and from each came a tantalizingly different aroma, as appealing as the odors of an old-time apothecary shop.

"Do many people around here practice herbal medicine?" I asked Clay

Anderson, editor and publisher of *The Ozarks Mountaineer*—a lively and informative monthly magazine keyed to the interests and activities of the region. "It would be hard to give a figure," he replied. "But there is definitely a certain continuity. Often grandparents did something with herbs, and passed on their recipes to their offspring, who continue to use them and pass them on.

"Not that many of our people try herbs for all their doctoring, or would know how if they wanted to. On the other hand, if they are products of this environment, which has limited resources, and where there have been few doctors and almost no hospitals, they have had to endure and to do for themselves. The natural thing would be to follow the ways of their forefathers. Also, when you live close to nature, you have a keen awareness of it. Everything—the plants and animals especially—makes you feel part of it, of a grand scheme. It's only reasonable, then, to think of natural curatives at hand to help you.

"Even some of our doctors may turn to herbal preparations for an old-fashioned patient; they ask, perhaps, if he has peppermint or yarrow growing in his yard for indigestion or a cold. Certainly you can say the Ozark people are not really returning to nature," Clay said. "They've been there all the time."

As I roamed the rolling highways and rutted dirt roads of the hill country, I met some of those Ozarkians who have never left the healing arms of Mother Nature.

There was Chick Allen, who owns the Wash Gibbs Free Museum and Country Store near Branson.

"I'm the fourth generation of my family hereabouts, and I'm part Delaware and Cherokee Indian," he said, as we sat on a little balcony near his Indian and Civil War exhibits. "I've been a farmer and a country musician in my time. I was a jig dancer, and I could get pretty good music from the jawbone of a mule."

Lean and lined, and as tart of word as one of his remedies, Chick Allen is the author of several informally written pamphlets. In subject, these range from the exploits of his grandfather in the Civil War and misdeeds of early Ozark outlaws to lists of herbal remedies used long before there were "store boughten" ones.

"During the Civil War, about all they had was bitters," he said, referring to any concoction made from bitter-tasting plants. "It wasn't till afterward that herbs were flavored to make them taste good."

In his booklet, *Ozark Root Digger,* Allen lists some 30 plants to treat various ailments: horsemint, for instance, for the common cold and to help quiet an upset stomach; elder bark to kill parasitic screwworms; wahoo for chills, fever, and malaria.

"The white man learned how to use these herbs and roots from the Indians," he wrote. "Many a life in the early frontier days was saved with these remedies. In the Spring . . . people gathered enough roots and herbs to do them until the next Spring. . . . time to shed their red underwear and to get their Corn Liquor Stills to running, because all good medicines contained some corn Whiskey for preservative."

I asked Chick Allen which plant he found the most useful in his concoctions. "I use more goldenseal than anything else," he answered, describing a short, hardy plant with greenish-white blossoms. "I make a tea with it or eat it dry. I recommend it as an eyewash. If you have a sore on your leg that won't heal, you can beat up some goldenseal and put it on the spot. It'll heal. You can also mix goldenseal with mutton tallow or soot from an old wood stove, and it makes one of the finest salves for humans or animals.

"Sassafras root is another good medicine. If you get a swelling in your legs and feet from being on them a lot, you can drink sassafras tea, and a nip of goldenseal, and it'll take the swelling out overnight. That's what the old-timers did.

"I'm an old-timer now, but the good Lord has been kind to me. I've hardly ever been sick even with a cough or a cold. I've done my own doctoring. If I needed something, I went into the woods and got it and cooked it up myself.

"Some of my children and grandchildren still dig herbs, but mostly they run to the drugstore. It's easy for them, but I remember when the closest hospital was Springfield, 15 hours away by horse and buggy. A lot of operations had to be done right in the home then. Babies, too, were all born there. My mother was a midwife, and a good one. Sometimes it was for a neighbor family, but often she had to travel all over."

Pushing on to the Ozark village of Walnut Shade, I visited a retired midwife — spry, 86-year-old Ella Ingenthron Dunn — who still gathers her own medicinal plants.

Mrs. Dunn, or "Aunt Ella" as she is called in the community, has published a small book entitled *The Granny Woman of the Hills*. A "granny woman" is a midwife, but Aunt Ella wasn't writing about herself; she was telling the story of her mother, who had been a midwife before her, and of the hardscrabble life of her homesteading family.

"In my time, I brought 71 babies into this world and never lost a one," Aunt Ella said proudly as we talked in her comfortable living-and-dining room. "I never had a bear cat either — that's what you call it when you can't handle a delivery.

"One little nine-pound boy did die — of strangling, I think — but that was before I could get there. On my way with the father, we hurried so fast that we never even stopped when a black cat ran across the road."

In 20 years of midwifery, Aunt Ella traveled "every way you can think of" to deliver babies, she said. "On foot, by muleback, horseback, horse and buggy, farm wagon, and by car. Calls often came at night, and sometimes we had to go 15 or 20 miles on a case," Aunt Ella continued. "Once it was eight degrees below zero when I got up from my warm bed and went out. Being a granny woman was more like an angel-of-mercy business than a job. Occasionally there was only a 'thank you,' and five dollars was all I ever got, except one time when I worked 16 hours, and they gave me ten dollars."

There were other rewards, however. As she leafed through her records, I noticed how her voice warmed up in speaking of friends and neighbors she had helped, and of the children she had delivered who came to visit her after they grew up.

When I asked Aunt Ella if she used herbs to treat ailing babies, she said she had found that a little goldenseal solution was good for an infant's sore mouth. Also I learned that granny women all carried a little black bag containing such things as catnip leaves and watermelon seeds, in addition to the traditional cotton, white muslin, scales, scissors, goose grease, camphor, and cornstarch.

In her book I read that a tiny amount of catnip tea was administered "to help the baby rest better," and that the watermelon seeds "were steeped in a cup of water and sweetened and given (1/4 teaspoonful) to work the kidneys if any trouble showed up in them."

Aunt Ella is also an ardent follower of natural medications for herself. "My kids occasionally tell me to get a prescription from the doctor," she said, "but I don't believe in pills. When I was growing up, we didn't have a doctor in the house till I was eight years old, and then only because my father caught typhoid fever.

"We did buy a few things, such as asafetida. Nearly everyone wore a little bag of asafetida around his neck then, mostly to calm the nerves. You could also take a little bit of it, the size of a lady pea, in water, and it was the best nerve medicine in the world. But even now, I like to dig in my garden, when I'm able to, for any medicine I need.

"This purple herb here is digitalis," she said, as she showed me some of her growing plants. "It's a good heart medicine, and it's pretty, too. I use the bark of the wild cherry tree over there for my spring tonic, and the roots of the mandrake — or mayapple plant — are good as a purgative when mixed with whiskey. And over there's my garlic. I use the buttons — the part of the bulb down in the ground — for high blood pressure.

"But you'll find all this in my new book," she added, "if I ever get time and help enough to write it. I wore out two dictionaries on the first one!"

Wherever I went, I asked Ozarkians about wild ginseng, partly because of the high price a pound brings today — $80 or more to the digger, and still more to the distributor.

"There's not much around here now," said one herb collector. "A couple of years ago, some men came in from outside and just about cleaned out most of it."

Unexpectedly, however, I ran into a bit of luck when I was referred to

Robert S. Prewitt of Spokane, Missouri. It turned out that he had a patch of ginseng growing in a deep gully on his extensive property. "This is a typical environment for it, dark and damp," he said, as he led the way down a long, steep hill to a clump of underbrush concealing a spring. "And we're fortunate today—there's one mature plant. You can tell it's ripe because of its red seeds. Over there is one that's still green. It usually takes five or six years for ginseng to mature," he added.

With his short, sharp knife, Mr. Prewitt dug a narrow hole several inches deep until he freed the fist-size root—the commercially precious part of this foot-high, delicately green plant. Because of its forked shape, which at maturity resembles a man's body, the Chinese named this root *jen shen,* or man plant.

"This is the wild variety," he said. "It's worth a lot more than the cultivated kind. But I don't dig it to sell. I just like to see it grow and spread.

"Sometimes I chew the root for its sweet flavor," he replied when I asked if he used it himself, "but my grandparents, who used many Ozark herbs, felt that it was a fine overall remedy. I've heard that people in Asia consider it a fertility drug and an aphrodisiac. Maybe that's because it increases energy and well-being in general."

I didn't know it then, but when I drove away, I carried not only the ginseng root that Mr. Prewitt generously gave me, but also other mementos from his thick underbrush. Such field souvenirs, namely ticks and chiggers, have been labeled "the wildlife of the Ozarks." I managed to get rid of the ticks, but the scores of chiggers that had attached themselves to me went along on my next visit to an exuberantly charming woman who has become the Ozarks' most famous herbalist—Billy Joe Tatum.

Though Billy Joe is not a professional botanist, she has spent 20 years studying wild flowers and herbal lore. She also writes regularly for *The Ozarks Mountaineer,* and has just published a best-selling cookbook and field guide on foraging for wild foods. Some reviewers of the book see her as Arkansas' successor to the nationally known herbalist and writer, the late Euell Gibbons.

One of my first questions when she took me on an herb-collecting trip through the meadows and woods near Melbourne, Arkansas, was, "Where can I find something to help my chigger bites?"

"We use pennyroyal," she said, pointing to a fuzzy-looking plant with many small leaves and branches. "We'll gather several bunches of it and boil them into a strong tea to splash on your bites." And that's what we did. I must confess that the decoction did not at once completely cure the inflammation. But I give it credit for easing the itch of the bites that drives some victims nearly mad.

From Billy Joe I learned, among other things, that jewelweed is another treatment for itch and rash; that slender leaf mountain mint helps an upset stomach and can mask bad-tasting medicine; and that she knows Ozarkians who smoke mullein leaves to relieve sinus congestion.

Asked to lunch at "Wildflower," Billy Joe's rambling wood-and-fieldstone home perched high on a bluff near Melbourne, I found dozens of field herbs hanging to dry from the rafters of her kitchen-dining room.

"I always try to keep a supply on hand," Billy Joe explained, "and they're handy here. If you have an ailment, you can't always go out and pick the herbs you need."

With her physician husband, Dr. Harold Tatum, Billy Joe often entertains at wild parties—that is, with a menu made up of items she collected in the field. At the luncheon for me, we had wild pheasant salad; chutney made of black haw berries, apples, and wild onions; apple and spearmint salad; elderberries that tasted like capers; iced sumac tea; and bread made of cattail pollen and whole wheat. Delicious!

As with others, I asked Billy Joe how widespread is the use of medicinal plants in the Ozarks. "There are a number of people who still prefer them," she said, "but nothing like as many as 50 years ago. Besides, it's hard, backbreaking work under a hot sun to dig these plants and then prepare them.

"As to the practice of herbal medicine among doctors around here, you'll have to talk to my husband. I know he gives a few prescriptions containing herbs. I myself was particularly interested in dittany as one to lower temperatures. One of the names people call it around here is fever plant. I experimented and discovered that three or four cups of dittany tea would reduce fever as quickly as ten grains of aspirin."

Dr. Tatum, I learned, agrees with his wife that professional medicine can benefit from the popular interest in returning to natural products. "I think it's a very refreshing trend," he said. "The only bone I would pick is that overenthusiastic lay people may think they can diagnose as well as anyone, and use herbs to treat the wrong disease.

"My young partner here, Dr. Craig Milam, gives herbal prescriptions if he feels his diagnosis warrants it, and has been quite pleased with the results. In fact, I understand that some doctors, especially those fellows out of medical school within the last five years or so, are choosing to work in rural areas like ours where herbs are available, instead of opting for more lucrative practice in conventional urban centers."

Deep in the hot, dusty hills in Belen, New Mexico—30 miles south of Albuquerque—I met Tibo Chavez, an herb enthusiast with a heritage completely different from that of Billy Joe Tatum. Mr. Chavez is a practicing attorney who served as a state senator for 20 years, and as lieutenant governor for two terms. But his passionate avocation is rooted in the hundreds of herbs, mostly medicinal plants, which he constantly collects, both in the wild and on his 200-acre farm.

This fascination with herbs is part of his overall interest in preserving the history and culture of New Mexico, and it reaches back to his Spanish family, which was one of the earliest to settle in the Southwest.

"As far as I know," said Tibo, "the original Chavez arrived with Juan de Oñate, who was an explorer and colonizer. He led an expedition into what's now New Mexico in 1598. In those days, and for many generations after, medical treatment meant brewing teas and mixing poultices and such from available plants. Even after the first doctors came here to the lower Rio Grande Valley in the late 1800's, many people distrusted their remedies. The few families who could afford to call in a physician often considered it a status symbol; some prepared their own prescriptions on the side with recipes inherited from ancestors.

"I myself grew up with herbs," said Tibo. "My mother used most of those I plan to show you. She always had jars and cans around filled with this and that herb. One of my earliest memories is of sipping a tea made from *manzanilla,* the 'little apple,' also known as chamomile. It was used for colic and other infant ailments.

"Gradually, herbs became a lost art in my family as the feeling grew, especially among the more educated and affluent, that it was just the poor and ignorant who clung to the old ways. It was not until I got into politics and went out into the country that my faith was revived by hearing of illnesses cured by herbs after doctors had failed. And also by my personal experience, for instance, in drinking *yerba buena,* a spearmint tea used to cure a stomachache.

"For years now, I've taken nothing but nature's medications. Some members of my family follow this example. My youngest son once had some pimples and used a salve made from comfrey, and the pimples went away. Even when I had a heart attack, I told my doctor that I would diet and take it easy, but that I would stick to herbs for my heart instead of swallowing his medicine.

"The doctor agreed that I looked fine, and later I took him a clump of *mastranzo,* or horehound, which he planted in his yard. Whether he ever uses it, I don't know, but I'm sure he wonders about my herbs."

So enthusiastic is Tibo Chavez about herbal medicine that he frequently gives talks on the subject at the University of New Mexico and elsewhere. He also has published an illustrated book on popular *remedios* of the area. He never makes specific suggestions for treatment, however. "I'm certainly no doctor," he says. "I just report on the history and usage of the plants.

"But we may be coming to the end of an era," he told me sadly. "Our old-time *curanderos* and *curanderas* — men and women healers — are getting along in years. We've got to visit them now, and see their herbs and way of life before it's too late."

With Tibo to introduce me to his friends, I met poor and well-to-do healers, Spanish-American, Indian, and Mexican-American healers, as well as garden-variety herbalists. And I saw and handled enough medicinal plants to stock a hospital.

"My son cut his hand on a piece of rusty barbed wire last week," said

Filemon Baca, a descendant of one of the first Spanish families to farm the area. "I made an ointment out of the leaves and roots of a *contra yerba*—a kind of thistle—and the wound cleared up without any infection."

At the small adobe home of Mrs. Alejandro Moya, the widow and inheritor of the curandero skill of her sheepherder husband, talk ranged from herbs and flowers that grow in the valleys to those that flourish only in the uplands.

The desert's *amole,* or yucca root, I learned, is made into a sudsy shampoo that eliminates dandruff. The lush, green *oshá* of the parsley family is a product of the mountains. "The oshá was a wonder plant to Alejandro Moya," Tibo remarked, "and still is to curanderos who can get it, and especially to highland sheepherders who consider it a medicine kit in itself. They chew the dry root for toothache, headache, and indigestion, make it into a poultice for sores, and boil it into a tea to treat a cold. They also drink it to prevent hangovers, and believe that the very presence of the plant keeps snakes away."

As usual on such visits, Tibo brought welcome gifts of cloth bags filled with herbs, and often received others in exchange. Indeed, so many plants were mentioned that it was hard to keep track of all the Spanish names and multiple uses.

For rheumatic pains, Mrs. Moya liked *estafiate,* Rocky Mountain sage, and *treto,* purple sagebrush, administered in hot baths. Tibo told of having suggested to an uncle suffering from severe arthritis a solution of *yerba de la vibora,* turpentine weed, in regular soakings.

"It worked so well," he said, "that my uncle's doctor asked for samples of the medicine to study."

The group, which included several members of the Moya family, spoke of using such *remedios* as *pague,* field marigold, for stomach trouble; *canutillo,* Mormon tea, for kidney and urinary disorders; *eneldo,* related to dill, for chest congestion; and *inmortal,* of the milkweed family, to ease childbirth.

As Tibo and I traveled about the countryside, I heard other stories of the healing power of "simples," as plant remedies used to be called. A tea decocted with saffron—more familiar to city dwellers as a food coloring and a flavoring agent—is commonly used in this part of the Southwest to treat measles and to lower fevers.

Anise, an ancient and favorite spice found in Spanish kitchens around the world, serves another purpose here in treating bad coughs. Pitch scraped from a piñon pine and made warm and gummy has long been applied as a poultice to bring a boil to a head or to extract a deeply imbedded splinter that has caused an infection. *(Continued on page 36)*

Overleaf: Spreading branches canopy a mountain springhouse in southern Virginia as Victoria Bowling adds water to a jar of freshly cut slippery elm bark. This gentle beverage—used by early pioneers—will aid digestion.

IRA BLOCK

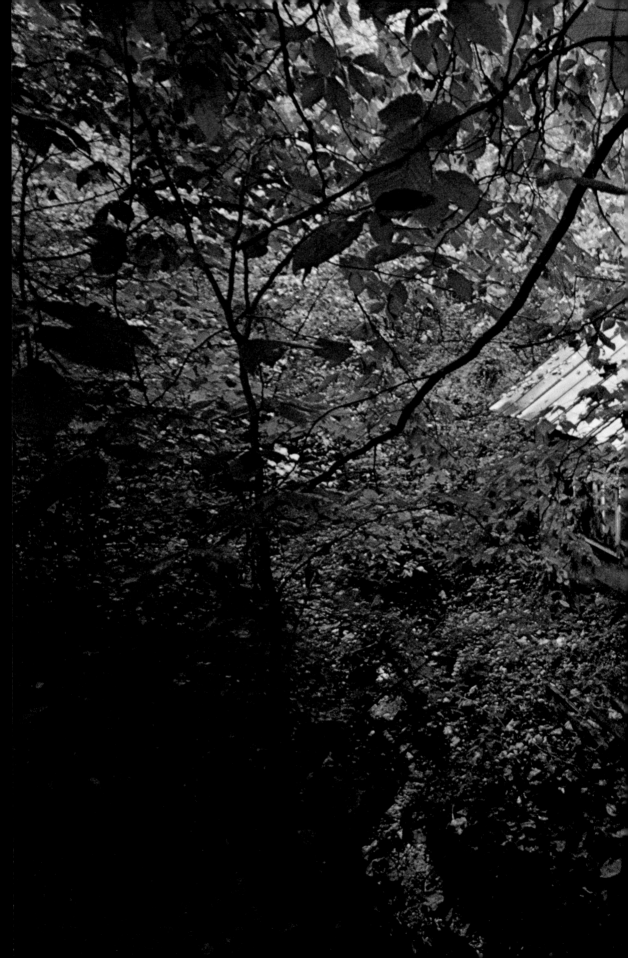

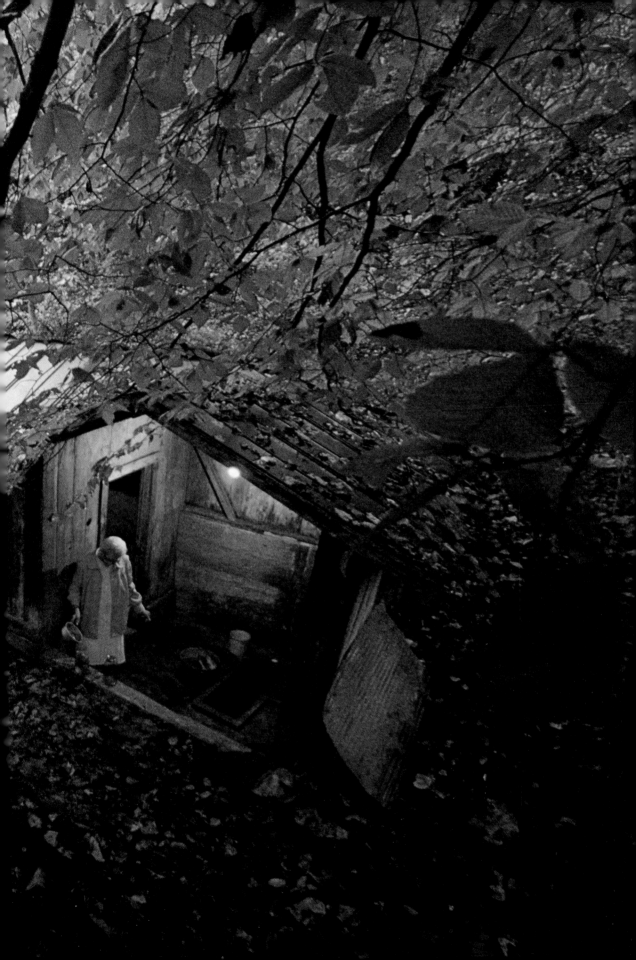

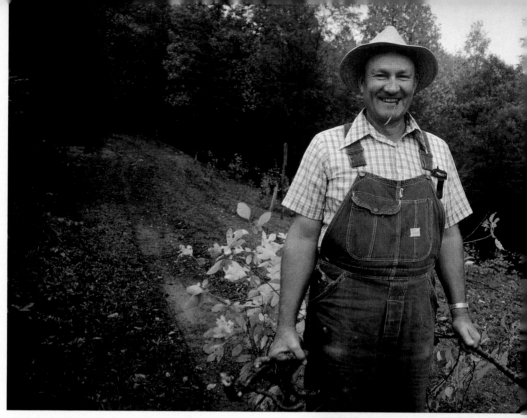

ALL BY IRA BLOCK

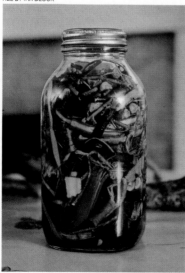

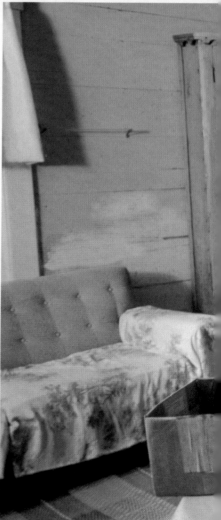

28

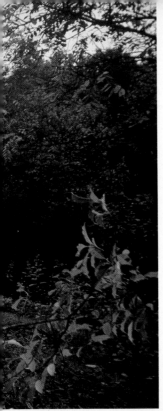

Hands full of healing plants, Wilton Nichols carries sassafras root and a branch of wild cherry gathered in the woodlands near Ferrum, Virginia. His mother, Victoria Bowling, mixes them with other roots and barks for a "good-for-what-ails-you" tonic (lower, left). As they combine the ingredients in her kitchen, Mrs. Bowling explains part of her recipe: "The cherry tree bark is for colds—it makes you sweat. I put bloodroot in to perk up your appetite, some sassafras for flavoring, then I sweet up the jars with honey and add grain liquor to charge up everything."

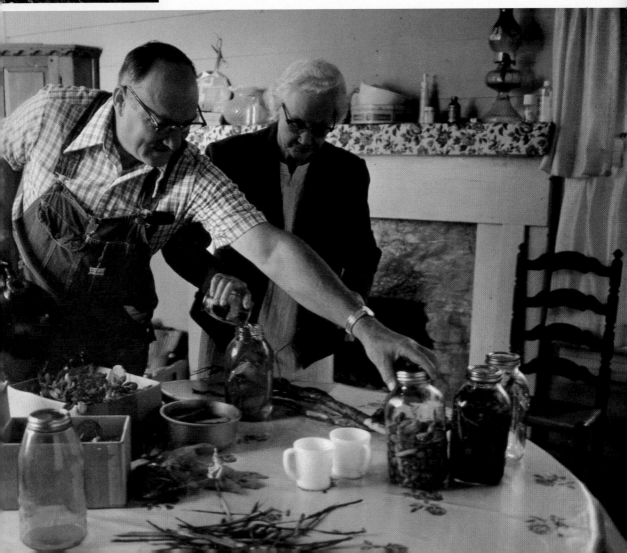

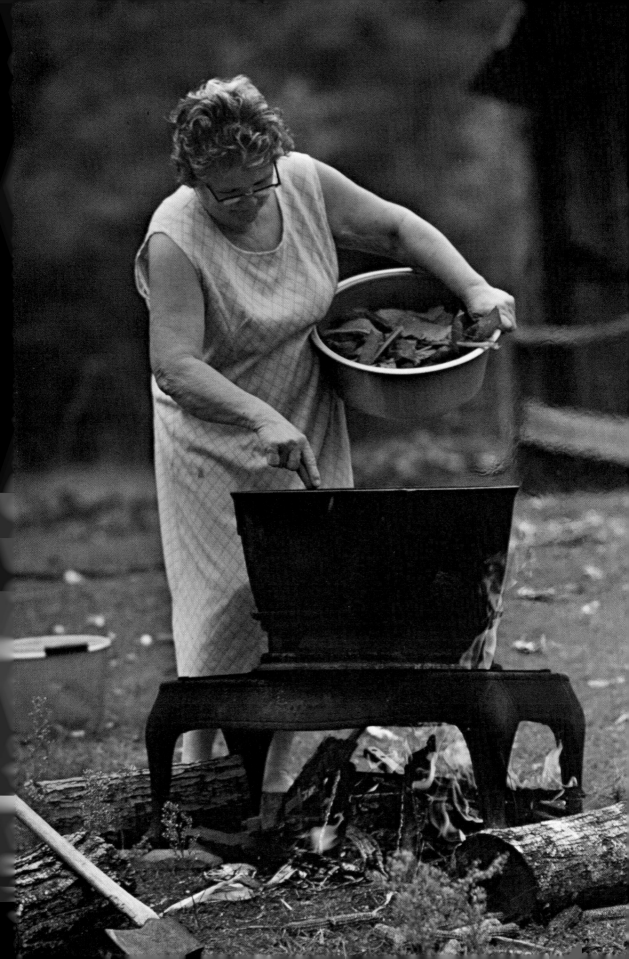

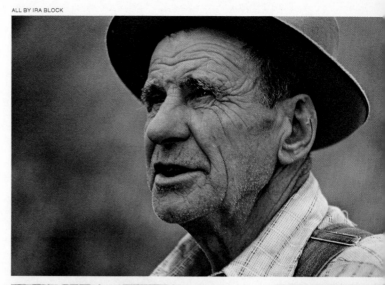

"I make my comfrey tea by boiling it down right good, that's all. It's nice and green when it's just right," says Ethel Radford. Outside her home near Floyd, Virginia, she stirs freshly picked comfrey leaves into a kettle of bubbling water, brewing a sweet tea for calming coughs and stomach ulcers. Her husband, Swanson (upper, right), an expert woodsman and beekeeper, helps her gather medicinal plants for the family. "Where we lived, we didn't go to doctors," says Mrs. Radford. "We dosed ourselves with the herbs all around us, and I think kids were healthier then than they are now." At right, she dips cups of the steaming tea for her grand-daughters, Linda and Jane.

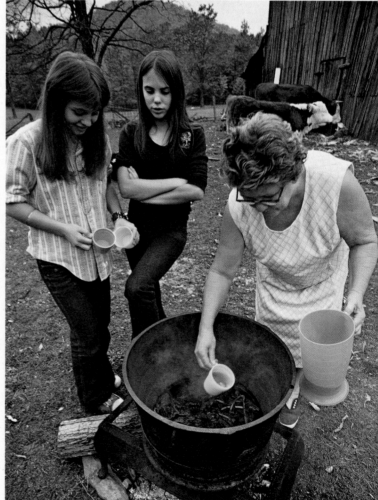

31

Nature's apothecary: Grinding comfrey, mint, and yarrow, herbalist Kathy Cranor blends the leaves and blossoms to mix with ginseng root for an invigorating tea. More than 175 different herbs and spices line the shelves of Pipsissewa Potions, her shop in Blacksburg, Virginia. "I spend a lot of time simply teaching their uses to customers," she explains. "But I try to caution people against experimenting with wild plants—you have to know what you're doing." Returning from a morning of foraging (below), she carries a mullein plant and a basket of its leaves.

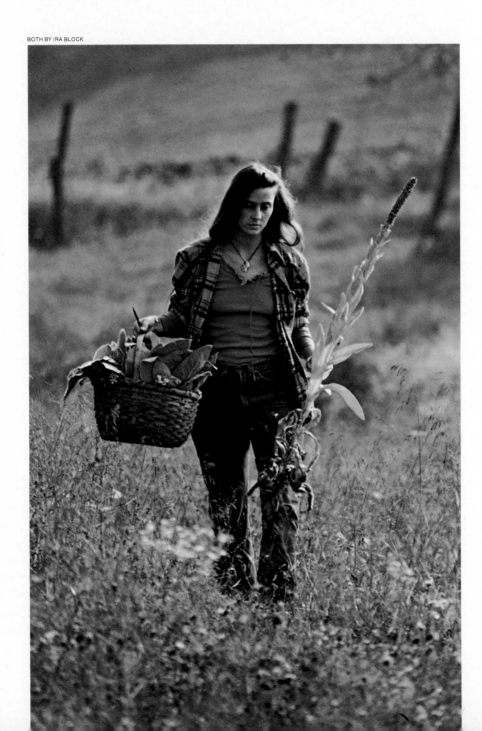

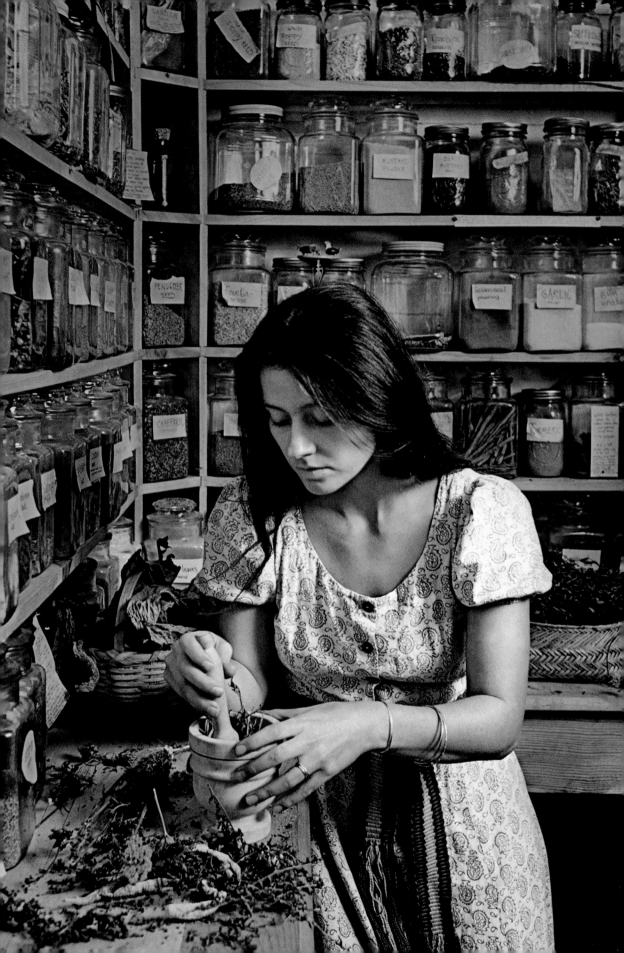

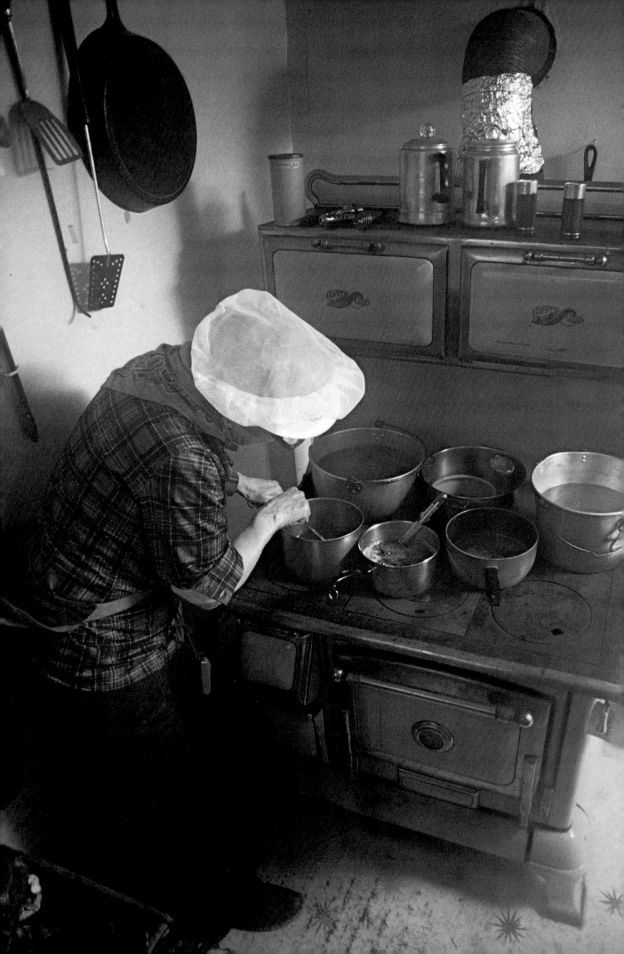

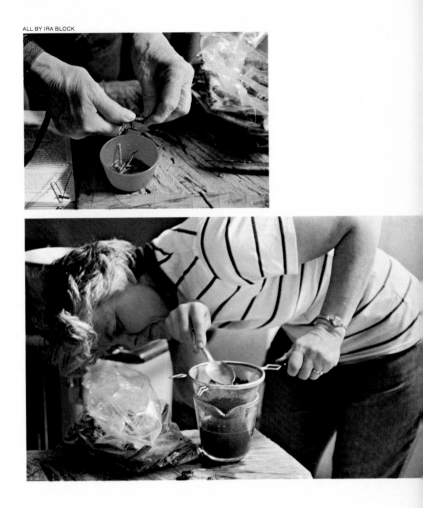

*Tantalizing blend of herbal aromas
fills a country kitchen as Ella Pfeiffer
stirs homemade cough syrup over a
wood-burning stove. As part of a
class given by the Audubon Naturalist
Society to interested city dwellers,
she prepares wild foods and natural
medicines at her instructor's farm
near Madison, Virginia. At top, she
cuts white pine twigs; with clover,
mullein, and wild cherry bark, they
form the base of her cough syrup.
After simmering fresh horehound
leaves, Portia Meares (above) strains
the flavored juice — the main ingredient
in a cough-lozenge recipe.*

Herb fanciers of the Albuquerque-Belen region of New Mexico do not buy commercial insecticides if they are bothered with house bugs or mosquitoes—the worst of the local pests. Dried leaves of a wild gourd called *calabasilla,* mixed with the prolific *barbasco,* or wild cinnamon, "will drive all the bugs—and mice too—right out of your house," said one of our hosts.

Another popular curandera, Mrs. Eufalia Otero of El Cerro, has patients who come from dozens of miles away, and pay eight dollars a visit for her treatments. Some have reported surprising results—of high blood pressure lowered, for instance, by drinking a liquid made from *mariola* of the aster family, or of sores healed by applying dried and ground leaves of the *yerba del manzo,* or lizard's-tail herb.

As with the conventional doctor, Mrs. Otero's stock-in-trade lies partly in her personality, which includes a ready smile and good-natured joking. "Here's where all my magic is," she said, bringing out a big bag of herbs, and opening her refrigerator to show us homemade medications from her own prescription of ground yerba buena, oshá, and other plants, mixed with soap and sulfur powder.

To me, one of the strangest of Mrs. Otero's medications is deer's blood, which she keeps in a glass jar in the refrigerator. She obtains the blood from butchers and hunters, and gives it in carefully measured doses for heart trouble. This practice presumably grew out of an old belief honoring the strength and nobility of the deer's heart.

In many areas of the Southwest, I met family and professional healers, who, like Mrs. Otero, use not only common herbal medicines, but also such strange substances as deer's blood; many of these would raise the eyebrows of any physician.

The most memorable prescription I encountered, and one long followed, came from a retired sheepherder, Manuel Castillo, who told us how he dealt with two broken legs that he suffered in an accident years before. His curandero obtained the skeleton of a dog and ground it into a fine powder that he browned in the oven. He then made a sticky plaster of it and smeared it on Castillo's legs, after the broken bones had been set and a splint applied.

"My legs soon healed straight and true," Mr. Castillo said, pulling up his pants legs to show us the proof. Some people might postulate that the calcium content of the dog's skeleton helped knit his bones.

Modern science does, indeed, explain the success of much folk medicine by the presence of helpful chemical substances found and identified in many plants and natural products. In other cases, doctors attribute the good results of earth-born treatment simply to psychological factors. Many cures, of course, combine a little of each. In the Southwest, four distinct cultures have mingled, each contributing its own dose of herbal lore and faith healing.

"When the Spaniards settled here, they brought their own medicinal plants, which have now been thoroughly interchanged with those of the native Indians," said Tibo Chavez as we drove north from Belen to visit some of his Tiwa Indian friends on the Isleta Reservation. "Later, with the opening of the Santa Fe Trail, came the contributions of the *Anglos,* which merged with the other two and with the remedies, lore, and plants that for centuries have been coming into our valley from the peoples of rural Mexico."

At Isleta, on land that covers the site of a village occupied long before the Spaniards arrived, I talked with Maria Salazar and Lupe Torres about tribal herbs, past and present.

"In my time, we all had our babies at home and used many natural products to keep our families healthy," said Mrs. Torres. "We would grind up twigs, berries, and dried leaves between a large flat rock and a rounded hand rock, then mix a poultice, or boil or steam the powder in water over hot stones. I used to tie up lots of little bundles of an herb we called the tea of the fields, then brew them for a general tonic."

The *yerba de la negrita* of the mallow family was given to mothers as a hot, cleansing drink after childbirth, she explained. It was good for diarrhea, too. Babies with sick stomachs were dosed with chamomile tea, and adults drank a liquid made from wild celery for their nerves.

"We also made cedar products into medicines for anything from treating sore throats and colds to easing girls' menstrual cramps," Mrs. Torres said. "I still use cedar for all kinds of things. During the flu scare last year we fumigated our house with smoke from branches burned in the fireplace. It made everything smell good."

Traveling southwest from Isleta into Arizona, I drove sunlit roads bordered by desert vegetation toward distant, misty-blue mountains. Nearly 70 miles southwest of Tucson, I came to Sells, the village headquarters of the Papago Tribe. Its reservation of more than four million acres covers some of the hottest and most arid land in the United States.

There I had arranged to meet Alice Norris, on the Executive Health Staff of the Tribal Government, who had promised to tell me something of the medicinal traditions and ways of the Papago people. It was a subject, I soon discovered, that was close to her heart; her Papago ancestors reach back to the days before the Spanish arrived.

A large and friendly woman with black hair piled high, she wore the symbol of her tribe on a silver necklace. "It shows the mysterious maze of life," she explained, pointing to the figure of a man surrounded by circles and incomplete lines. "It means there are things we can never know, but must accept.

"Every tribe has its own beliefs," she went on. "You probably have yours that you follow. We have simply continued to practice many of the things we did before there were doctors. We also believe that divine power is given to certain individuals who can cure illnesses and even cast out evil spirits. The Bible says that Moses was told to do some remarkable things, and he was able to do them."

As we talked, I learned that there are a number of practicing medicine men and women on the Papago Reservation. Patients usually go to them for treatment, but, in the case of a very ill patient, the medicine man may make house calls—if he is provided transportation.

The way the system operates is both complex and precise, as much as when conventional doctors accept patients and set up tests, consultations, and treatment. "There are three types of Papago medicine men who work together as a team," Alice said. "There is the diagnostician, the singer, and the herbalist. Sometimes, if you think you know what's wrong, you go directly to the herbalist. But generally you see the diagnostician first. He doesn't examine in the usual sense. He simply talks with the patient; he sings, or chants, certain verses depending on how serious the illness is, and he meditates for a while until the condition is revealed to him. Then he sends the sick person to a second medicine man—or occasionally a woman—who also sings with the patient and performs the specific remedy recommended by the diagnostician.

"If the patient is still not cured, the final step is to go to the herbalist, who prescribes plant medicine for the ailment. I was very sick recently, but I only had to see the first two medicine men." The story Alice Norris told me was a fascinating one. She was in Phoenix attending the National Conference on Aging when she became so ill with nausea and fever that she had to return home to the reservation. She saw a medical doctor there, who prescribed medication, but it did her no good. "I was thirsty, but I couldn't swallow," Alice recalled. "So a diagnostician was brought in to talk to me.

"He referred me to a singer, who said there was something in my throat that had to come out. After the customary ceremony, he put a tissue on my neck. Then he put his lips to the tissue and sucked very hard. When he raised his mouth, he showed me what he had drawn out—an object known only to a medicine man, covered with a kind of mucus. He said I would feel very weak the next day but be well enough.

"After he left," she concluded, "I drank some water and ate two small bowls of chicken rice soup. The next day I was sore, but, just as he predicted, I felt well."

Later, Alice took me to see her friend, an elderly medicine man named Sam Angelo, in his neat little house at the end of a long, dusty road. Although blind, he carries on a successful and highly respected career on the Papago Reservation.

It was hard to remember that he was blind as we sat and talked of his work in a room decorated with religious paintings and carvings. In his crisp, blue-striped shirt and blue cotton pants, his voice strong and serene, he seemed to be in complete control of his environment.

Sam does not limit himself to purely ritual treatment, I learned after he showed me his special charm—a small, worn figure of a horned toad, carved without horns to represent his own blindness. He uses herbal substances as well.

Speaking in the Papago language, translated for me by Alice, he mentioned some of the medicinal plants I had seen and heard about in New Mexico: yucca roots, mashed and boiled to make a tea for treating diabetes, and mountain oshá, the all-purpose sheepherder remedy recommended so highly by Tibo Chavez.

In fact, Sam Angelo had just returned from a trip to administer oshá medication to a woman in another Papago village. The patient was apparently suffering from some kind of stomach disorder, and Sam remained at her house for four days to provide the required dosages of the healing herb. It was "to clear her insides," he explained.

Before leaving the Papago Reservation, I visited the Indian Hospital of the U. S. Public Health Service, where, I had been informed, professionally trained physicians work frequently in conjunction with Indian medicine men in caring for their patients. "That's hospital policy," said the tall, thin, young director, Dr. Tim Fleming. "If a patient feels there is more to his illness than can be treated by means we provide, and if he or his family wants to call in a medicine man, we're glad to cooperate. The hospital is always open to the traditional healers for diagnosis or treatment, day or night.

"I've lived with five different Indian nations in the past few years," Dr. Fleming said. "I have a high respect for these people, and I have a special interest in making this hospital more available to traditional medicine. The power the medicine men have is not easily documented or appreciated by all our doctors. We must walk carefully so we won't destroy the benefits that they can bring to the Indian patients."

I was surprised to find Indian healers working side by side with physicians using modern medical techniques. But I was even more surprised to discover the full extent to which folk medicine is practiced throughout the United States. Nearly everyone I met had some pet remedy—passed down through the family—that supposedly cures or alleviates some ailment. And nowhere, I found, is folk medicine more popular than in the Appalachian Mountains—one of America's leading herb-using and distributing regions.

"From the hollows and hillsides of the Appalachians, many plants have been spread to other sections of the United States," said Dr. James A. Duke, chief botanist at the Plant Taxonomy Laboratory of the Department of Agriculture in Beltsville, Maryland. "Goldenseal and ginseng are good examples. Ginseng grows especially well in Wisconsin."

To consult an Appalachian-born student of folkways and herb medicine, I drove from Washington, D. C., to the home of Earl Palmer in Christiansburg, a small town in southwestern Virginia.

Mr. Palmer, a country naturalist and free-lance photographer, was the town's mayor for five terms, and is now a bank director there. He has walked the mountain trails of Appalachia all his life, and knows the people well who live in such communities as Turkey Cock, Raven's Den, Rock Castle, Joint Crack, and Runnet Bag.

"Self-sufficient mountain folk," he calls them, "who keep to the customs of their ancestors, and make do with what they have. Boiling herbs comes as natural to them as moonshining, which still goes on around here. So do the same old 'revenooer' raids and shotgun 'feudin's' between rivals in the business.

"Mixing moonshine whiskey with herbs comes natural, too," he said. "One of the teas they call bitters is made with whiskey and ratsbane, bloodroot, ginseng, pokeberry, and honey, plus wild cherry, sassafras, and slippery elm bark. In the past, the whiskey was brewed right on the home place and contained only pure grain alcohol. It was considered an all-around tonic, and was a common inhabitant of many a family's medicine shelf, on tap for assorted ailings—including those times when you're 'feeling poorly' or just 'tollable.' "

As we drove and walked about the hill country, Earl pointed out his favorite trees and herbs, and described how Appalachian families use them. "Take yellowroot," he said. "It's one of the first herbs to flower in March, about the same time as blue violets. When cut and broken, yellow-root produces a very bitter, orange-red juice. And there's nothing better than a round of bitters to jack up a feller a notch or two and get him out to plowing after a winter of laying around the house.

"Many of the herbs found hereabouts help cure coughs and colds by making you sweat," he continued. "'That pretty goldenrod, cooked up into a hot tea, is one of them. Another is boneset, which you generally find along creeks and in damp woodlands. It's particularly good for fever and flu. Then there's pokeroot — a valuable plant for all kinds of ailments, from rheumatism to the itch. And the barks of several trees are useful, too. When I was a boy and had a sore mouth, my mother would get the inner bark of white or black oak and boil it into an astringent dose that would soon fix me up.

"In fact, I agree exactly with the herb gatherer who once told me, 'T'aint nothing what grows ain't good for something.' "

With Earl Palmer as guide, I rode one Sunday morning across three mountain ranges to visit Roy Blackwell. "The best ginseng hunter in these mountains," Palmer calls him.

Parked in Mr. Blackwell's front yard were the two jeeps in which he prowls the hills. Soon we were admiring his latest haul, a collection of ginseng roots gathered on a four-day trip to Haycock Mountain, towering on the hazy horizon above Wood's Gap.

Spread out on the ground and drying in the sun on a long sheet of aluminum was more ginseng, of all shapes and sizes, than I had ever expected to see in one place. "This batch is nearly dry," said Mr. Blackwell, "and weighs about a fourth of what it did when the roots were green. The older roots are more valuable than younger ones because they're supposed to get stronger with age. You can tell the difference by the number of markings on the rhizome, the stem at the top of the root. It's like telling a tree's age by trunk rings added each year."

I asked Mr. Blackwell if he uses ginseng to treat himself, and he replied that he occasionally chews a little for indigestion, but that mostly he gathers it for sale.

"There's a good market for it," he added. "Ginseng's said to be good for just about everything you can think of."

At another stop on our travels in the mountains, we waited for the return from church of a couple reared in these parts, and who still follow many of the old-time customs. Invited to visit with Ethel and Swanson Radford, we sat on a pleasant, plant-decorated front porch and talked about nature's bounty and how to use it.

"Where we lived, we didn't go to doctors," said Mrs. Radford. "I didn't need to when I was growing up. We dosed ourselves with the herbs all around us, and I think kids were healthier then than they are now. I raised my own family that way, too. When the babies were fretful, a little warm catnip tea soothed them, and we made a fine cough medicine for croup from honey, vinegar, and alum. For fever we boiled up teas from snakeroot or from spicewood branches. Horehound was good to keep the kidneys working, and there was nothing like sassafras tea in the spring to pep you up.

"We still make many of these teas, and some are as good for animals as for people," she said. "When I was sick before my gall bladder operation, I got relief from a tea made with the broad leaves of that comfrey stand you see across the road. I also splashed some of the same stuff, good and hot, on the wounds of one of our pigs after a horse stepped on it. It's almost well now."

But I remember best something else Mrs. Radford said when we talked about the honey they gather from a cluster of bee stands set up in an apple orchard near the house.

"Honey is condensed herbs," she said, "and it's good for the whole body. I love the bees," she added, her kind, motherly face alight. "I go around talking to them, and to the flowers and to the birds, too. No matter what people say, I know they know me."

Driving back to Washington from Christiansburg, I thought of other nature lovers and folklorists who are preserving the knowledge of lingering ways of life and "herbing" in many places. In Rabun Gap, Georgia, deep in the rolling hills of the southernmost Appalachians, a remarkable project began in the 1960's, when Eliot Wigginton, a young high-school teacher, launched his class on a magazine-publishing venture.

The name chosen by the students for their magazine was *Foxfire*, after the glow given off in the dark by decaying wood; their objective was to record the thoughts, customs, and activities of the region's mountain people before it became too late.

So eager were the youngsters about their magazine that they raised the money for the entire project themselves, and soon began collecting material through interviews with parents and grandparents, and by field trips to rustic cabins in hidden coves and valleys. Putting together all of their tapes and photographs, they issued the first edition of *Foxfire* — 600 copies in March 1967.

Since then, several of Eliot Wigginton's classes have worked and graduated, but new ones keep the magazine's glow bright for a circulation that has now reached nearly 5,000 in the United States and in several foreign countries.

Three large books have been published from the enterprise, with yet another in the making, and several hundred high schools and other groups are following Rabun Gap's example — from Maine to California, from Minnesota to Mississippi, and also in the Virgin Islands, the Dominican Republic, Alaska, and Hawaii.

Foxfire itself has more than fulfilled its original purpose. In quarterly issues, it has shown how hill people continue many of the region's early American customs — often under hardship, but with the compensation of sturdy independence through nature's bounty. Quoting old-timers in mountaineer words and cadence, the youthful reporters of *Foxfire* have saved from oblivion many old recipes, superstitions, pithy sayings, and home remedies. Straight from the mouths of convinced users have come these treatments:

"For arthritis, make a tea from either the seeds or leaves of alfalfa. . . . Place a spiderweb across a wound. . . . For diarrhea, drink a little blackberry juice."

If you have a cough or sore throat, "eat a mixture of honey and vinegar," or swallow a syrup made with wild cherry and other barks, or "make a tea from the leaves of boneset. Drink the tea when it has cooled. It will make you sick if taken hot," they warn.

Less convincing, but more entertaining, are other beliefs reported by *Foxfire:* "To cure cramps," goes one, "turn your shoes upside down before going to bed." Or to remove a sty on your eyelid, "run it over with the tip of a black cat's tail."

My favorite remedy, however, deals with a tapeworm. "First you starve it," the sufferer is advised. "Then you hold some warm milk up to your nose and sniff deeply. The tapeworm will stick his head out of your nose. . . . Hold the milk farther and farther away from him, thus drawing him out."

This last suggestion, I suspect, is mountain humor. But in all such lore, I've found, there is a mixture of the practical and the preposterous.

Some herbal concoctions are obviously worthless. Others may be harmful or even fatal. But many have won enough support from satisfied customers to become standbys in folk medicine everywhere.

In a little Vermont town more than 60 years ago, a young doctor named DeForest Clinton Jarvis began studying and experimenting with the natural medicines of country people in his state. So impressed was he by many of the herbs and other substances used that he adopted them for his own practice. In 1958, he published a best-seller called *Folk Medicine* that described his experiences with patients and his resolute belief in the efficacy of Vermont lore. It is now in its 21st printing.

In his book, Dr. Jarvis discussed the body's need for minerals and vitamins found in the same wild greens that people pick in the Ozarks and other places I had visited—dock, dandelion, anise, catnip, and peppermint, among others.

He also suggested the consumption of kelp, a seaweed, for its mineral content. For external uses, he relied on the age-old remedy of castor oil, a favorite of the ancient Egyptians. Applying it to moles, warts, and skin ulcers, he said, would remove or lessen these blemishes. Applying it to hair and eyelashes would make them more luxuriant. And mixing castor oil with turpentine, and then rubbing it liberally on the chest would alleviate a cold or bronchitis.

But the theme song of Dr. Jarvis's folk medicine carries the steady beat of honey and apple-cider vinegar, a pair of home remedies I frequently ran across on my travels.

To the Vermont doctor, honey and vinegar—whether taken together or separately, internally or externally—offer ready answers to problems ranging from coughs, burns, and bed-wetting (honey) to shingles, food poisoning, and varicose veins (apple-cider vinegar).

All over the United States, you can find other pockets of folk healing like those of Vermont.

"The majority of urbanites think of the use of plants and other natural products for self-medication as a quaint custom of the past," wrote Julia F. Morton in a book published in 1973 called *Folk Remedies of the Low Country*. "The truth is that in many parts of the world, . . . even in the centers of bustling cities, folk medicine is a living art and a *normal* way of life for millions of people."

Dr. Morton, director of the Morton Collectanea—a botanical library at the University of Miami—names and describes scores of plants that provide the only medicines of a rural community made up mostly of Gullahs and descendants of other African peoples living off the land in the low country of South Carolina, near Charleston.

Many plants she lists, such as Virginia snakeroot and calamus, or sweet flag, are common ingredients of folk medicine elsewhere. Others have special pertinence here.

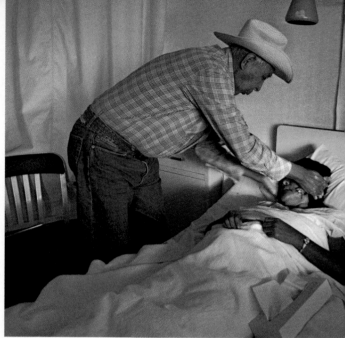

With gentle touch and soft chants, Papago medicine man Sam Angelo helps ease a patient's pain. When requested, this blind healer visits Indians at the reservation hospital in Sells, Arizona. Such medicine men cooperate with staff physicians, who recognize the effectiveness of their traditional medicine.

Life everlasting is an astringent herb particularly prized by both city and rural folk in this part of South Carolina as effective against flu, diarrhea, mouth ulcers, and other sores and wounds. Each fall, bundles of its dried, blossom-topped stems are still transported to the Charleston City Market and sold there in large quantities.

Dr. Morton also found pomegranate, chinaberry, and wormseed among plants of the Gullah people that have additional historical and medical interest. Introduced originally from Africa and the Caribbean, they often went into the medicine chests of southern plantations to treat the family and slaves.

"When I was on North Caicos Island in the Bahamas," she told me, "I heard some of the very same medical expressions—'check your stomach up' was one—that I encountered in the South Carolina low country. The duplication suggests an intriguing link with the time when Colonial planters often held estates and slaves in both places."

Euell Gibbons, whose enthusiastic pursuit of the plants he fondly called "wildings" made him the leading popular herbalist of our time, was impressed with the medicinal folklore of his Pennsylvania Dutch neighbors. He especially admired their many uses of catnip, "the herb that makes cats ecstatic."

They drink cold catnip tea as a tonic before meals, he noted in his book, *Stalking the Healthful Herbs*, and for relief from gas when served hot afterward.

"When any member of the family gets a cold, or the flu, he is put to bed, covered warmly, and given hot Catnip Tea with lemon," Gibbons wrote. "This is said to induce copious sweating, lower the fever, and help break up the cold. . . . It is doubtful that this treatment ever measurably shortens or actually cures any cold," the author admits, "but it does make the patient more comfortable and helps him to rest, and I defy any cold medicine to do more."

As I continued to seek information, I was amazed at the number of people I met who look back with nostalgia on home remedies practiced on them by their mothers and grandmothers. Florian Thayn, a Washington colleague, once told me how her Western Mormon heritage included such cures as a mixture of turpentine and honey that brought blessed relief to a croup sufferer.

"Sap from a pine tree was a common treatment for boils," she said. "When one desperate relative had tried everything else, milk was heated with lead pellets from a shotgun shell. It was strained and consumed by the victim, who never had any more boils.

"One of my earliest memories," said Florian, "goes back to the time when my brother and I picked up an 'itch' at our country school. To my fastidious mother this was a sure sign of a character flaw. But grandmother suggested the remedy of sulfur and lard. Never will I forget the night we stood on the dining room table and were slathered with this smelly concoction, dressed in our pajamas, and sent to bed. As I tried to sleep, I wondered if the itch or I would smother first. But somehow it worked—the next day the itch was gone."

For a professional opinion on the subject, I talked with Dr. Duncan Emrich, Professor of Folklore at American University in Washington, D.C. "I'm convinced," he said, "that every family in the United States has at least one cure for its ills. I once asked my radio listeners to send me any family remedies they had for diseases or afflictions. They came in from every state in the Union."

In his book, *Folklore on the American Land*, Dr. Emrich quotes many of these replies, including some as fantastic as a cure for quinsy—an inflammation of the throat. It called for filling a double thickness of flannel with live earthworms, and pinning it around the neck of the sick person for a specified time.

But all such cures cannot be lightly dismissed, he observed. "As in the cases of moldy bread preceding penicillin and the psychogenic nature of wart cures, the medical profession discovered in 1882 that the principal arachnidan isolated from spider webs proved in pill form an excellent . . . remedy for malarial fever and ague. A folk cure which had seemed wholly idiotic and useless prior to this medical discovery was a pill rolled from whole spider webs."

That popular interest in folk medicine is not only continuing but also growing can be seen firsthand in the multiplying natural-food stores that are springing up all over the United States.

It's almost as if nature were fighting back against the encroachments of modern civilization and technology by speaking ever louder to those people with ears close enough to the ground to catch the clues to her long-hidden mysteries.

Hoping to relieve a headache with the aroma of nicotine, Remedios Moya of Valencia, New Mexico, places revenue stamps from cigarette packages on her nose. When her brother-in-law, Manuel Castillo (below), broke both his legs, a curandero, *or healer, set his fractures and applied a sticky plaster of ground, baked dog bones. "My legs healed straight and true," he said. Like other Spanish-Americans in the Southwest, Mrs. Moya and Mr. Castillo practice the traditional medicine of their ancestors.*

BOTH BY NATHAN BENN

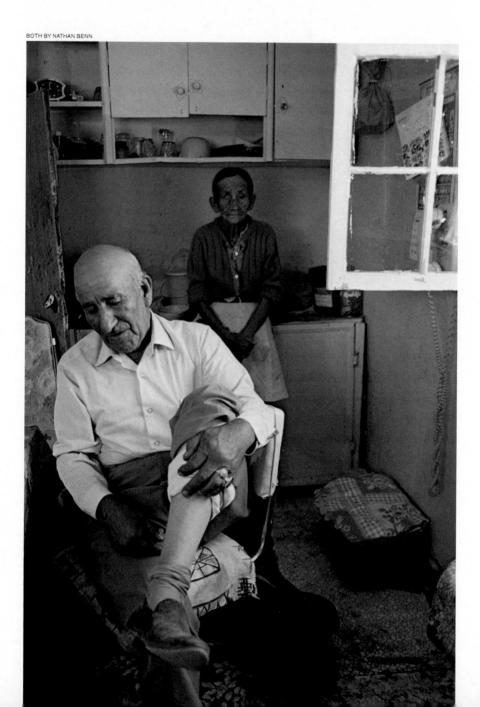

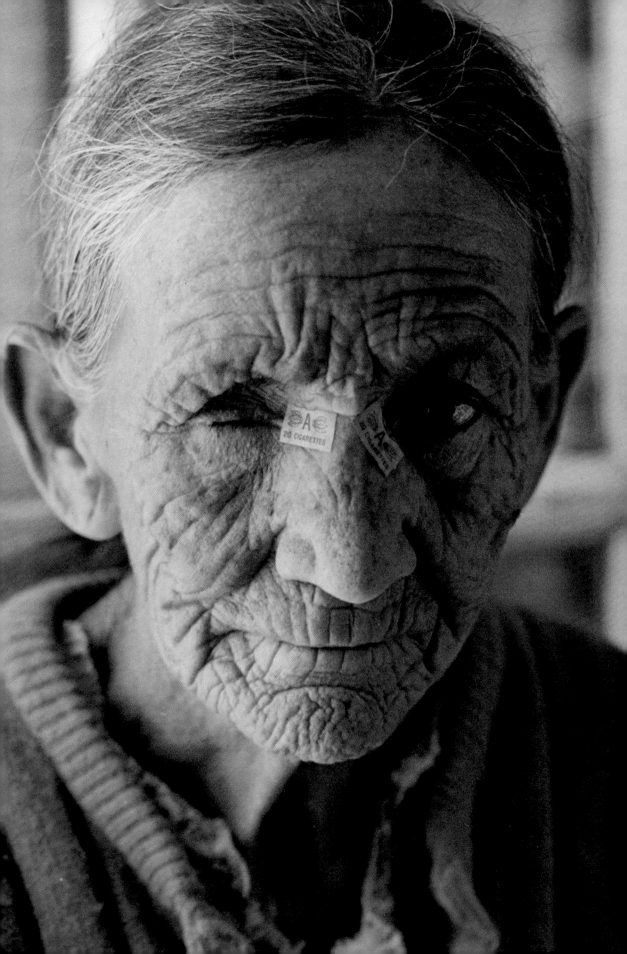

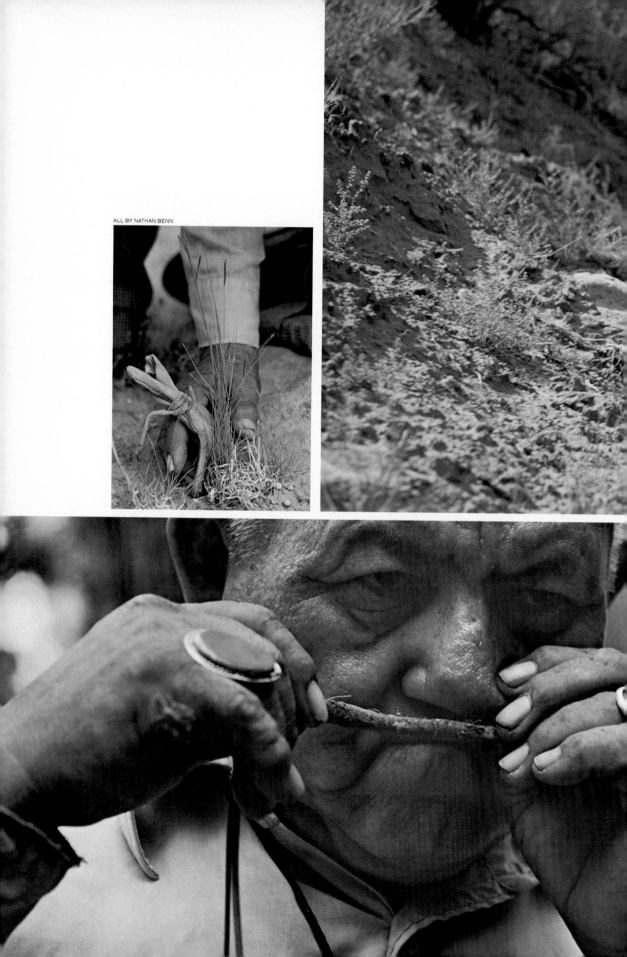
ALL BY NATHAN BENN

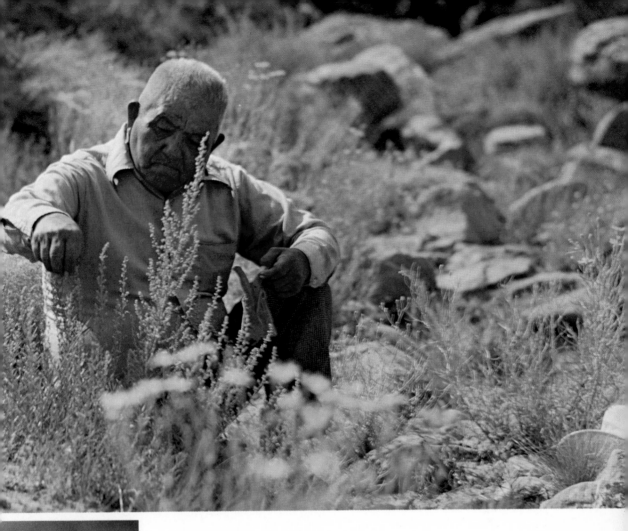

Performing an age-old Navajo ritual, medicine man Ray Winnie sprinkles corn pollen on a cliss rose as an offering to the plant. After blessing this cliss rose— which will remain untouched—the medicine man collects others of the species. In the Lukachukai Mountains of Arizona, Navajo Indians still gather sacred herbs for ceremonial and medicinal use. Above, left, Ray Winnie holds his corn pollen bag against a clump of grama grass—one of the seven basic herbs in Navajo belief. To identify the oshá plant, he sniffs the root (left), known for its pungent odor. Both Indian and Spanish-American healers use oshá to treat coughs and colds—and to keep snakes away.

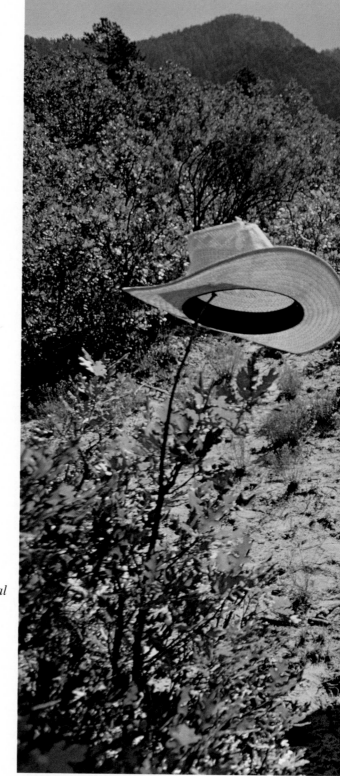
NATHAN BENN

Listening to Ray Winnie's melodic chanting, two students from the Navajo Community College watch quietly as he makes an offering to a mountain mahogany plant. To learn more about Navajo culture and tribal lore, they accompanied the medicine man on a field trip to collect herbs. Skilled in Navajo oral tradition and herb usage, Ray Winnie serves as a resource aide at the college, sharing his knowledge with young Indian students.

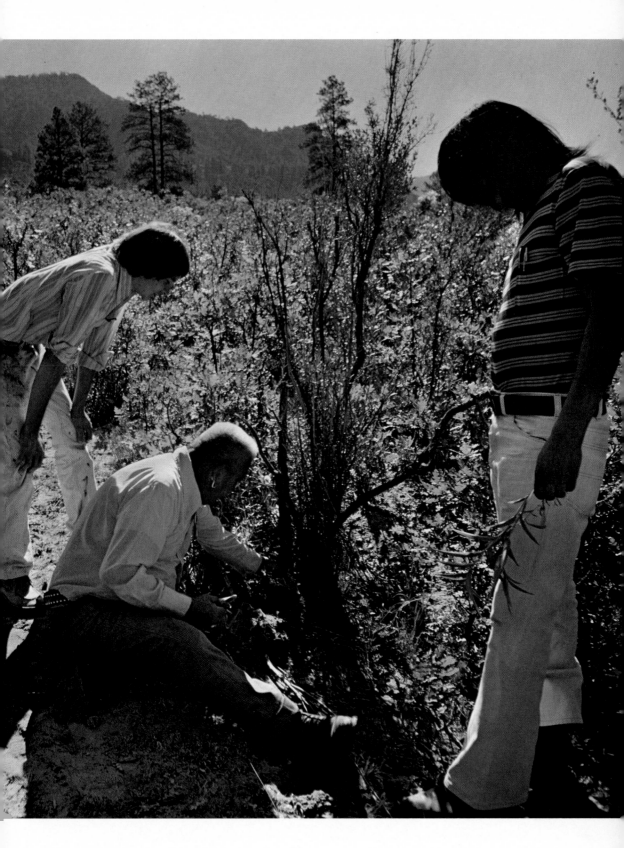

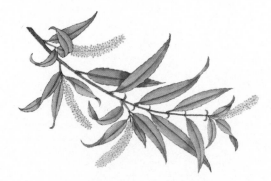

Legacies From the Past

THERE'S A SECRET INGREDIENT in every natural product found in each of the thousands of health-food shops scattered across the country. The ingredient is hope—at times called faith—that the wisdom and power of Mother Nature will ease that stomachache, heal that wound, and somehow make that pain go away.

Kennedy's Natural Foods in Falls Church, Virginia, is no exception. Ten years ago, Jim and Elinor Kennedy opened their market—one of the first all-natural-products stores in the Washington, D. C., area.

The idea began, they told me as we sat in their office above the store, with a pastor who had a serious allergy, and with his specialist, Dr. Theron Randolph of Chicago. The minister referred Mr. Kennedy, also an allergy sufferer, to Dr. Randolph, and out of this association and others with patients similarly affected, came the idea of a shop that would offer safe, natural products to customers plagued with allergies.

"At that time I knew so little about herbs and such that I didn't even know that a rose had hips," said Mrs. Kennedy, a slim, vigorous woman. "Luckily we had help selecting stock from a grocer named Walter Camp, who had grown up in Germany and was familiar with the health-food

"Glorious path over the mountains is rich with herbs," proclaims a sign at a Taiwan pharmacy. Like many peoples, the Chinese still rely on age-old remedies; a basket holds milk vetch roots—used in an invigorating tonic.

WILLOW (ABOVE)

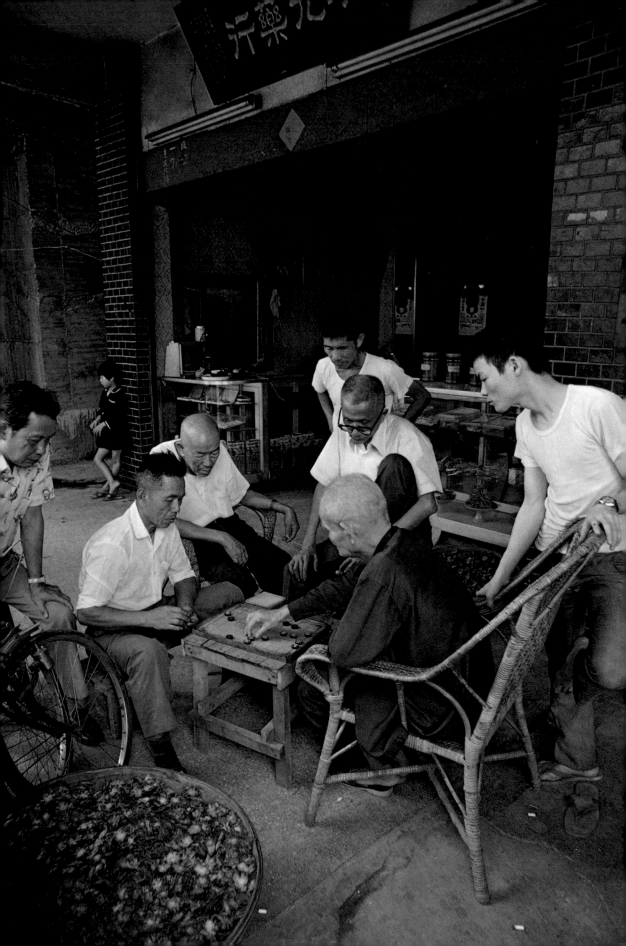

stores there. The original Kennedy store and its three other suburban counterparts differ from most such establishments in their anti-allergy orientation and strict emphasis on all-natural products. Everything they sell is organically grown, or produced without chemical additives or chemical feeding. Meat, for instance, includes such delicacies as ground elephant patties and reindeer and hippopotamus steaks.

Particularly interesting to me were the neatly boxed and bottled herb teas made from plants I had seen growing in wild and cultivated states. I found pennyroyal, with which I had doused my chigger bites in the Ozarks, and chamomile, the fragrant herb that Tibo Chavez's mother gave him as a colicky infant. I also saw desert yucca that the blind healer of the Papago Tribe in Arizona had used to treat his patient's stomach trouble, and comfrey that helped heal the wound a careless horse had inflicted on Mrs. Radford's pig in the Appalachians.

"We've come a long way since they called our place the 'Falls Church nut shop,' " said Mrs. Kennedy with a smile. "It's especially rewarding to me to provide sick people with natural diets and herb remedies that are prescribed by doctors.

"I remember the case of one woman whose family was about to have her committed to a mental institution. She had grown enormously fat and would often throw off all her clothes in a frenzy. Her allergist finally discovered that chemicals were driving her into the attacks. When she turned to cotton instead of synthetic clothing and to prescribed natural foods, she lost her excess weight and became rational."

Today, some psychiatrists and other physicians agree with pioneering allergist Randolph that allergenic substances absorbed by highly susceptible people may cause conditions diagnosed as hyperactivity in children, or hysteria, depression, and schizophrenia in older people.

"I can only tell you what I know about," said Mrs. Kennedy. "There was a boy hereabouts who was so agitated that his father was considering an institution for him. After hospital observation proved that his trouble stemmed from food coloring, additives, and other chemicals, a special diet without these substances brought him back to normal."

Some people regard the current popularity of such back-to-nature projects as a passing fad. Others patronize the health stores regularly, and win converts to the movement with evangelical zeal.

To judge for myself what these shops offer customers, I visited one or more in every city or town to which my travels took me. I found, of course, big and little ones, frowsy and elegant ones. But all shared common denominators, especially in medicinal herbs. I saw many of the same boxes and bags of herbal teas—catnip, yarrow, and sweet flag, for instance. There were earthen crocks of ground licorice, dandelion and sarsaparilla roots, dried pumpkin and sunflower seeds. I could buy asafetida pills and cooking and medicinal oils—avocado, safflower, and a vegetable oil containing garlic capsules. Papaya was available dried, sliced in syrup, or as a liquid concentrate. Ginseng, that ancient Oriental remedy for what ails you, could be had in a multitude of forms: tea bags, capsules, chewing gum, and the dried root itself.

For people who prefer to grow their own, there were potted herbs by the dozen, including such old-time favorites as lavender, fennel, and rosemary—plus a popular newcomer, *Aloe vera*. Several of my friends keep this succulent green plant on hand as a living medicinal salve. Cut one of its leaves, they say, and it exudes a clear jelly that eases the pain of a burn and promotes quick healing. Commercial firms produce a sunburn lotion from the aloe, which the Bible mentions as an ingredient used to prepare the body of Christ—and which physicians prescribe today for nuclear and other radiation burns.

Finally, nearly all health stores display collections of colorfully decorated books and pamphlets that give the histories of, and recipes for, various home remedies. In fact, this supplemental literature is a significant feature of the nature-and-health phenomenon, since the sellers of natural foods and herbs have no license to diagnose or treat illness. These books tell which products have been found helpful for certain ailments. The buyer, however, must always beware of self-medication.

Dr. Ara Der Marderosian, professor of pharmacognosy at the Philadelphia College of Pharmacy and Science, accompanied me to some of that city's health-food stores, and later spoke of the hazards of careless dosing. "There's nothing inherently wrong, of course, in promoting natural substances," he said. "Many old-country remedies were really quite good—so good, in fact, that trained chemists and other scientists are going back to the plant kingdom to investigate, fully and systematically, its medical potential.

"The trouble comes when people don't realize that we've learned a lot in recent decades about the pharmacology, chemistry, and toxicity of what goes into medicines, whether natural or synthetic. When you try to heal yourself with different herbal teas, for example, it's important to know exactly what you're cooking with. And if you drink too much of them, or mix them with other potent drug substances, you may end up poisoning yourself.

"There are other dangers, too," he continued. "People today seldom have practical knowledge—such as their grandparents gained from experience—of just how much of a product to use. Or they may fail to keep it refrigerated and let dangerous bacteria invade it. Meantime, even if the home remedy is harmless, the condition it's supposedly curing could be getting worse without proper diagnosis and treatment."

At the time of my visit to the Philadelphia College of Pharmacy and Science—the nation's first such institution when it was founded in 1821— there was a special exhibit of historical equipment, paintings, and other paraphernalia from the art of pharmacy.

It was a fascinating show, filling room after room with assorted mortars and pestles, odd-shaped apothecary jars, hand-cranked pill rollers, international prescription books, and hundreds of other devices used by pharmacists of the past.

I particularly enjoyed the display on the patent-medicine era of American history, when a gullible public fell under the spell of freewheeling pitchmen. Along the walls stretched extravagant advertisements for 19th-century nostrums, which make claims of today's drug promoters sound like modest understatements. Hamlin's Wizard Oil, for one, "cures all pain in man or beast."

Illustrating the florid text and testimonials from pleased customers, drawings and photographs depicted angelic little girls and sturdy barefoot boys, happy mothers holding perfect babies, and virile husbands welcoming back "Lost Manhood," thanks to Dr. William Raphael's "Galvanic Love Powders."

One huckster's ad, printed beside a rustic scene of carefree children at play, described the product as "The 'Joy' Remedy, Nature's Life Preserver, The Medical Discovery of the Age." It was "made from Pure Wild Honey, an Extract of Pine, and a Natural Gum." The remedy, it continued, has "performed the most ASTONISHING CURES in cases of Consumption, Asthma, Coughs, Bronchitis, and Chronic Lung Diseases. . . ."

The first medicine patent in the United States, I learned, was issued in 1796 to Samuel Lee, Jr., of Windham, Connecticut. That was only three years after the young Republic had passed a law offering patents to inventors under the Constitutional provision to advance the "Progress of Science and useful Arts."

Lee's patent protected what he labeled simply "Bilious Pills," later said to contain a potent mixture of aloes, soap, nitrate of potassium, and gamboge—a gum resin from Southeast Asia.

Other pill makers followed with patents for surprisingly similar bilious treatments. Like Lee's product, they were marketed as sure cures for anything from yellow fever and dropsy to worms and "female complaints." Although relatively few purveyors of the early prescriptions bothered to seek patent protection, the medical boom was on, and gradually spread over the expanding nation.

Traveling in brightly painted wagons, itinerant peddlers stopped for one-night stands in towns blossoming along new railroads. They offered old Indian remedies, "pried" from medicine men or beautiful Indian maidens, and warmed with firewater. They sold not only health but also entertainment, which, in its heyday, included performing animals, magicians, rodeos, and dancing girls.

The great patent-medicine era, however, spiraled into a decline around the beginning of the 20th century. Concerned physicians, druggists, and newspapermen joined forces to protest the sale of drugs containing useless and often harmful ingredients, such as abrasive chemicals,

"It's important that our students know the source of modern drugs so that they can relate them back to nature," says Dr. Ara Der Marderosian of the Philadelphia College of Pharmacy and Science. Lecturing on Securinega, a plant that yields a nerve stimulant, he teaches pharmacognosy—the science that deals with natural-product sources for drugs.

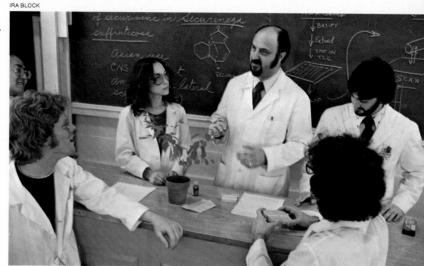

cheap liquor, opium, and cocaine. In 1906, Congress passed the first Pure Food and Drug Act, requiring a manufacturer's label and the names and amounts of all ingredients.

Of the few respectable products that remain from that flamboyant period, perhaps the most famous is Lydia E. Pinkham's Vegetable Compound. Advertised in the 1880's as a "Positive Cure for Female Weakness," it is now more modestly sold as a medication "to help relieve . . . that 'Too Tired' feeling . . . and other discomforts of 'Change of Life.' " Its ingredients are still all nature's—Jamaica dogwood, pleurisy root, licorice, and iron.

After showing me the historical exhibits, Dr. Der Marderosian took me to his college's modern laboratories and introduced me to several of his students. "One of our class projects," he explained, "is to collect, analyze, and report on herbs and other substances bought in various health stores, or extracted by chemical processes from plants grown in our own research gardens.

"In the last couple of years," said Dr. Der Marderosian, "we've also been looking into the exotic herb and animal products sold in the Chinese section of Philadelphia. When possible I give these assignments to my students of Chinese descent, because they can translate the labels. They follow the usual procedure of identifying a remedy's active component by its precise scientific name, then looking up past uses to see how it has rated as a medicinal application."

In search of some of the oldest medicines that students of pharmacognosy encounter, I visited New York City's bustling Chinatown, in a maze of narrow, winding streets in lower Manhattan. I was hoping to discover there a few of the ingredients listed in the earliest known pharmacopoeia —a book describing drugs, their preparations, and their uses. The *Pen*

Ts'ao, translated as *Essential Herbs,* is attributed to China's legendary God of Farming, Shen Nung.

Since Shen Nung is supposed to have lived nearly 2,700 years before Christ, any physical evidence of his work has long been lost. The names of his plants and other natural substances live on, however, in the records of later scholars, and especially in the 52-volume encyclopedia, *Pen Ts'ao Kang-mu,* which was compiled and published in the 16th century by the still highly respected physician-naturalist, Li Shih-chen.

I was thus happily surprised when I discovered in a single Chinese herb shop not just a few, but scores of substances that have been part of traditional Chinese medicine through the ages. In that small, neat shop, owned by a Chinese couple, Dr. Fook Kuan Lo and her husband, Dr. Woon Lam Ng—pronounced "Wu" in the Cantonese dialect—I saw hundreds of apothecary jars. Filled with powders, roots, and dried bits and pieces of all kinds, they were banked on shelves along the walls. Beneath the shelves, row after row of built-in wooden drawers, each divided into compartments, opened to reveal hundreds of additional products. Nearby, small packages with colorful Chinese labels held still more.

Besides their herbs, many of which belong to the same species I had encountered in the Ozarks and elsewhere, the owners showed me various animal parts. There was the velvet-surfaced antler of a young deer to be sliced paper-thin and combined with dried seahorses and herbs to make an "antler tea," valued as a general tonic. It also is prescribed to strengthen mothers after childbirth.

I gazed on snakeskin and thin strips of cattle skin used to treat human skin disorders, and the viscera of a frog that eases chest congestion when taken in a soup. A piece of rock-hard tiger bone would be ground into a powder and mixed with other materials for a poultice to heal injured tissues surrounding a broken bone. And tiger testicles were available for a potion to promote energy and virility.

Such animal medications may seem bizarre to Westerners. But in the 1930's, an American chemist and his associates isolated the hormone cortisone—which some then believed to be a miracle cure for arthritis—from the adrenal glands of slaughtered cattle. The animal extract was later replaced by a plant source, a Mexican yam, and cortisone itself did not live up to its first extravagant promise. But it is still a valuable drug that opened a new era in medical history.

Drs. Lo and Ng were both born in mainland China, but they met and were married in Hong Kong while studying traditional Chinese medicine. They received licenses to practice there, then moved to New York in 1967 and set up their own shop.

During my stay of several hours at their store, a steady stream of customers and patients came and went. From prescriptions signed by Dr. Lo and other Chinese physicians, the clerk behind the counter weighed out small piles of shredded and ground ingredients to be decocted or otherwise prepared at home. One set of eight different products used for headaches included mint leaves, sedge, buckthorn berries, cinnamon, orange peel, and licorice, peony, and ginger roots.

A young Chinese couple brought in their little boy, who had acquired two black eyes and a bruised forehead in a bad fall. Dr. Ng swabbed the injuries with a lotion of camphor and angelica as the youngster wailed loudly, then tentatively smiled through his tears, and finally munched contentedly on a cookie.

I learned more about China's ancient — and modern — arts of healing when another practitioner of traditional Chinese medicine, Dr. T. M. Pao of Lisle, Illinois, visited the National Geographic's headquarters in Washington. Dr. Pao, who left mainland China for Taiwan shortly before the Communist takeover, and who came from there to the United States in 1960, practices both herbal medicine and acupuncture — the ancient Chinese method of healing that uses thin metal needles inserted into specific points of the body. He lectures on health foods as well, and gives seminars on acupuncture techniques.

At the Geographic, Dr. Pao showed me more than 40 samples of the vegetable, animal, and mineral products with which he prepares prescriptions for his own patients and fills orders for shipment to various Chinese herb shops.

He imports all his raw materials from the People's Republic of China by way of Hong Kong, he said. He also follows the old Chinese practice of mixing different ingredients for the same prescription depending on the age and sex of the patient, and the season of the year.

One tonic for women called *Tan Kwe* reminded me of Lydia Pinkham's famous Vegetable Compound for ladies' complaints. In the Chinese version, however, something else is added. Mixed with its plant ingredients is a gluey substance extracted from boiled donkey skin — a remedy that goes back to the legendary Shen Nung, and which was described by Li Shih-chen as helpful in improving the blood and in regulating excessive menstrual flow.

To make a rejuvenating tonic for men, Dr. Pao imports considerable amounts of red ginseng roots. Most of his supply comes from Manchuria, he says, where the plant grows in abundance, with roots of excellent quality. The Russians use Siberian ginseng, also considered of high quality. American ginseng belongs to the same botanical family as the Chinese, but Pao finds its roots a bit rougher in appearance; he thinks that it is especially suited for skin problems.

Still, whatever its origin and quality, *(Continued on page 68)*

Overleaf: Cherokee herbalist bathes the ulcerated leg of a North Carolina planter with a decoction of sassafras bark; he will then apply a poultice of powdered maize and turkey down. Accounts such as this one from a colonist's journal of 1737 show how American settlers often relied on Indian medicine.

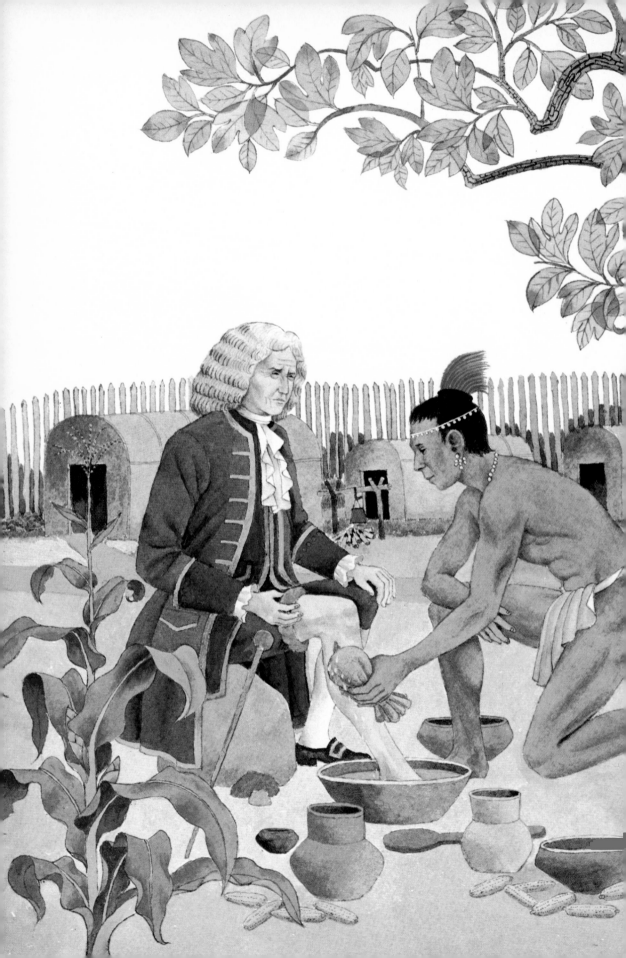

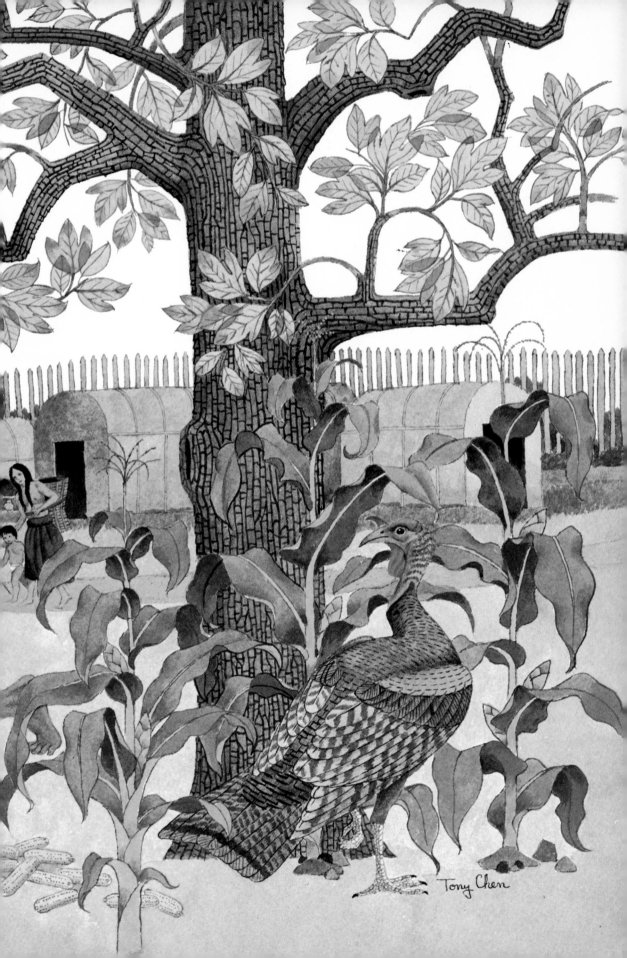
Tony Chen

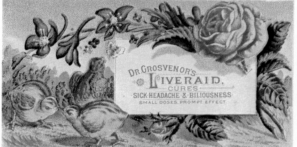

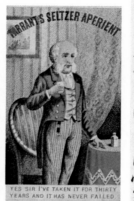

YES SIR I'VE TAKEN IT FOR THIRTY
YEARS AND IT HAS NEVER FAILED

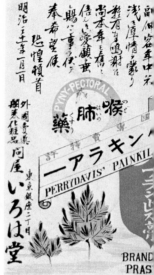

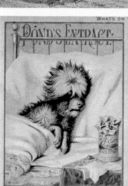

Advertisements and potions evoke the
colorful era of patent medicines, when

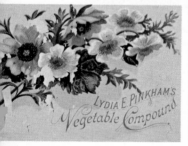

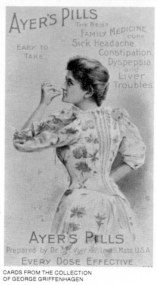

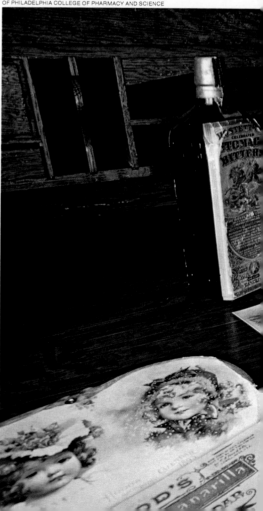

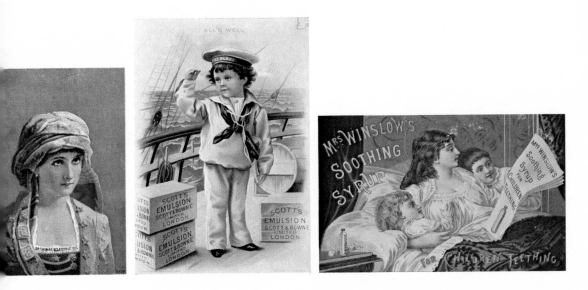

traveling hucksters sold suspect — and often harmful — medications. Distributed widely in various languages, 19th-century advertising cards extolled these "wonder cures."

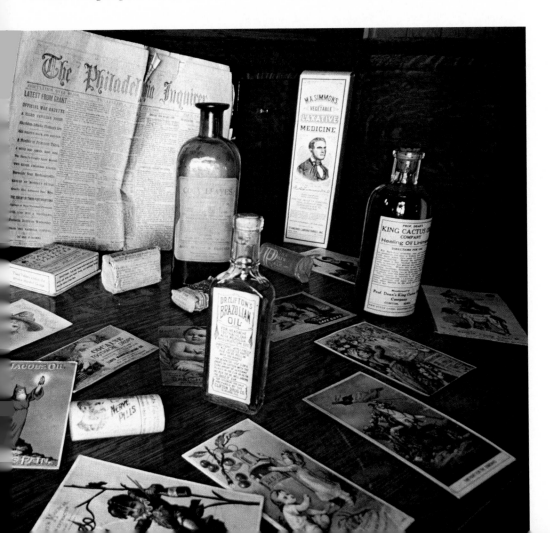

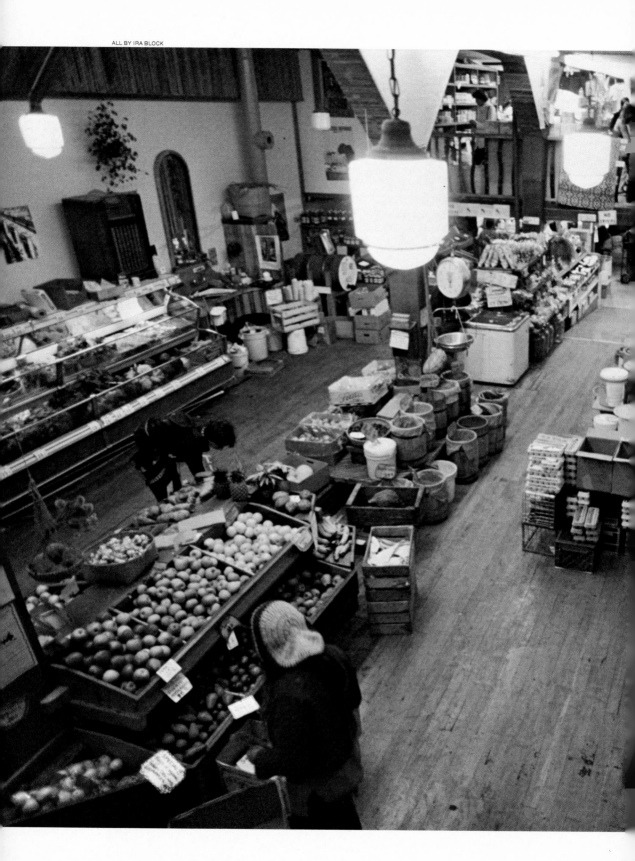

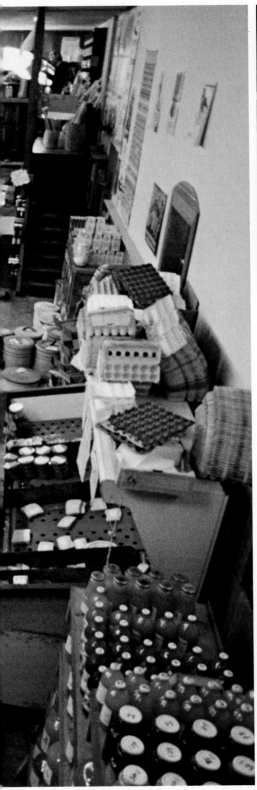

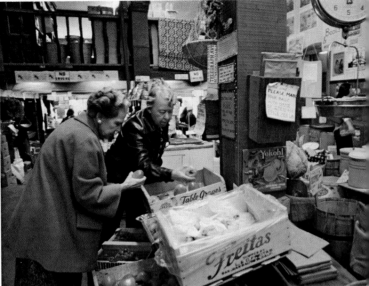

High ceilings and expanses of
hardwood flooring create a simple
spaciousness at Ma Revolution, a
health-food store in Berkeley,
California, that provides fresh
organic produce and bulk food.
Above, shoppers examine ripe
persimmons; below, crocks and
barrels hold several varieties of
rice. "People shop at health-food
stores," says employee Bruce Rice,
"because they realize that what
they eat affects how they feel."

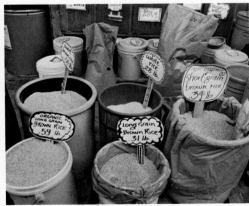

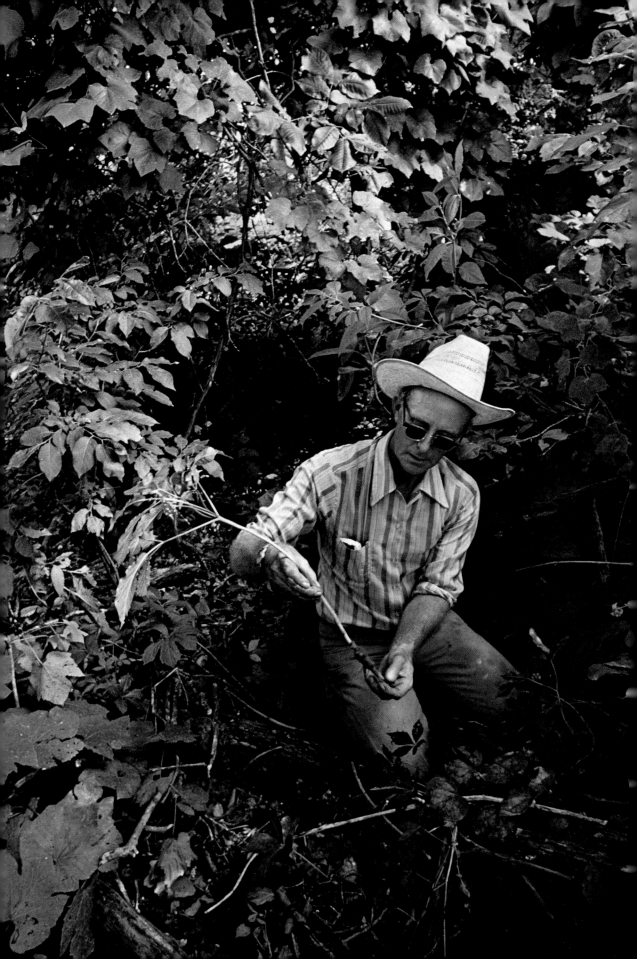

Moist black soil yields a wild ginseng plant to Robert Prewitt on his farm near Spokane, Missouri. "It's beautiful," he says. Exotic, elusive, and expensive, ginseng has helped remedy such debilitating diseases as anemia and has been taken as an aphrodisiac for thousands of years in the Orient. At right, Roy Blackwell of Floyd, Virginia, dries ginseng root in the back of an old car. He will soon replant the red seeds. Roy sells his ginseng to Hardy Palmer (below), an herb dealer in Christiansburg, Virginia, for an average price of $80 a pound.

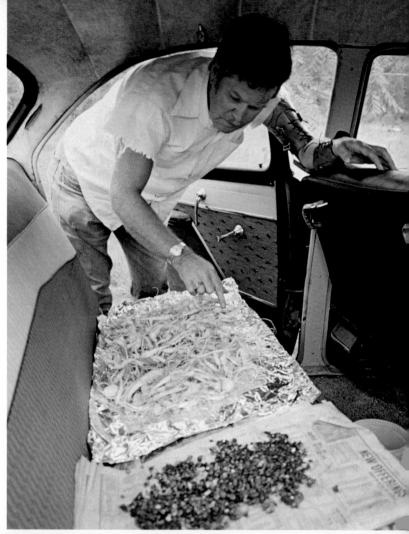

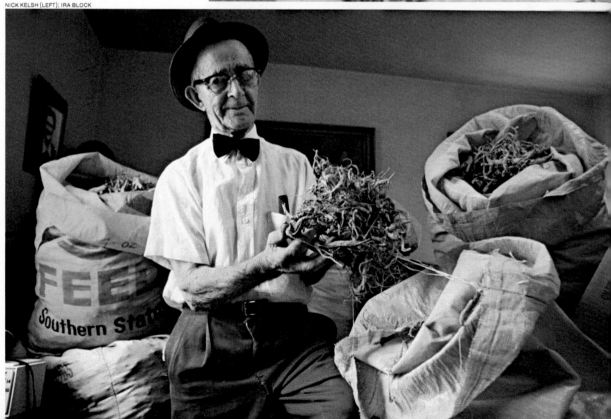

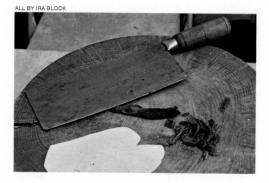

"I began drinking ginseng tea 40 years ago to recover from the flu, and I've hardly been ill since," says Harry Jew of San Francisco. To make the tea, he first slices white fook sung (left), and then boils it in water; he pours the resulting liquid over red ginseng root in a porcelain pot, secures the lid (right), and steams it for eight hours.

ginseng has captured the imagination of people, especially the Chinese, for thousands of years. More than 500 years before the birth of Christ, Confucius spoke of the healing power of this plant, and Li Shih-chen gave ginseng extra space and ardent praise in his erudite, carefully researched encyclopedia. "It would," he wrote, "allay fear, expel evil effluvia, brighten the eye, open up the heart, benefit the understanding, and if taken for some time it will invigorate the body and prolong life."

Another admirer had expressed a more specific and succinct opinion in India's ancient medical book, the *Atharva Veda*. "Ginseng causes an aroused man," he declared, "to exhale fire-like heat."

Though the Orient has never lost faith in the herb, Canada and the United States — the only other parts of the world to which it is indigenous — have seen its prospects rise and wane in medical and financial history. After word of the plant's powers spread from China to Europe in the late 1600's, French explorers discovered it growing wild in Canada, thus setting off a boom based on the hope of rich exports. Meanwhile, American colonists were finding their own wild ginseng supplies from New England to the southern Appalachians. Some settlers learned of the root's medicinal uses from Indians, who not only made it into teas to banish fatigue and treat illness, but also mixed it with several other herbs to form a love potion.

Other colonists, especially among the more educated and affluent, were inspired to try ginseng medications by reading of miraculous results described by the Chinese. William Byrd II, wealthy planter, writer, and political leader of Virginia, chewed the roots for years, and recommended the habit to his friends as a source of good health and long life. Byrd, who was born in 1674, lived to the age of 70 years.

The first boom in U. S. ginseng trade with the Far East began in 1783

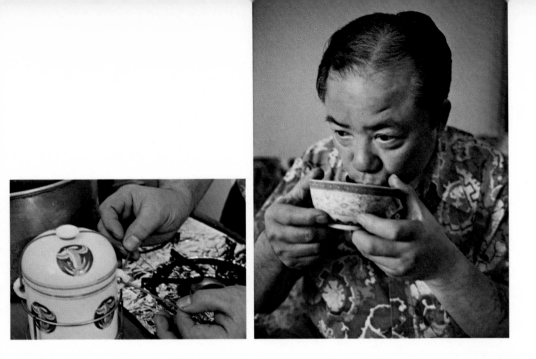

when an American sloop called *The Harriet* carried a small cargo of roots from Boston to China. In 1784, *The Empress of China* unloaded nearly 60,000 pounds of the increasingly valuable commodity in Canton. That same year George Washington, visiting his land holdings west of the Appalachians, recorded in his diary: "passing over the Mountains I met numbers of Persons and Pack horses going in with Ginseng. . . ."

By 1877, U. S. exports amounted to some $700,000, and enterprising New York farmers were successfully cultivating the wild herb under wilderness conditions of shade and moisture. Other planters cashed in on the new method until a fungus blight attacked the crops in 1904, causing bankruptcy and dashing many expectations of sudden riches.

Today, a new boom is under way, as ginseng products of all kinds are sold throughout the world, and popular demand for more threatens to make the plant an endangered species.

Even Western scientists are joining their Asian colleagues in taking a second look at claims made for ginseng as a universal panacea. Chemical analysis has long shown that the plant's roots contain minerals and vitamins, plus medically active constituents called saponins by chemists. Now half a dozen countries—England, France, Germany, Russia, South Korea, and Japan—are conducting research to determine just what effect these active substances have.

So far, investigations have produced evidence that drugs derived from ginseng roots can, indeed, strengthen and tone up the system, increase the body's resistance to stress, and *(Continued on page 76)*

Overleaf: Chinese physician-naturalist Li Shih-chen studies a broad-leafed rhubarb plant near Rain Lake in China. In 1578, he published an illustrated 52-volume encyclopedia of natural drugs and their uses.

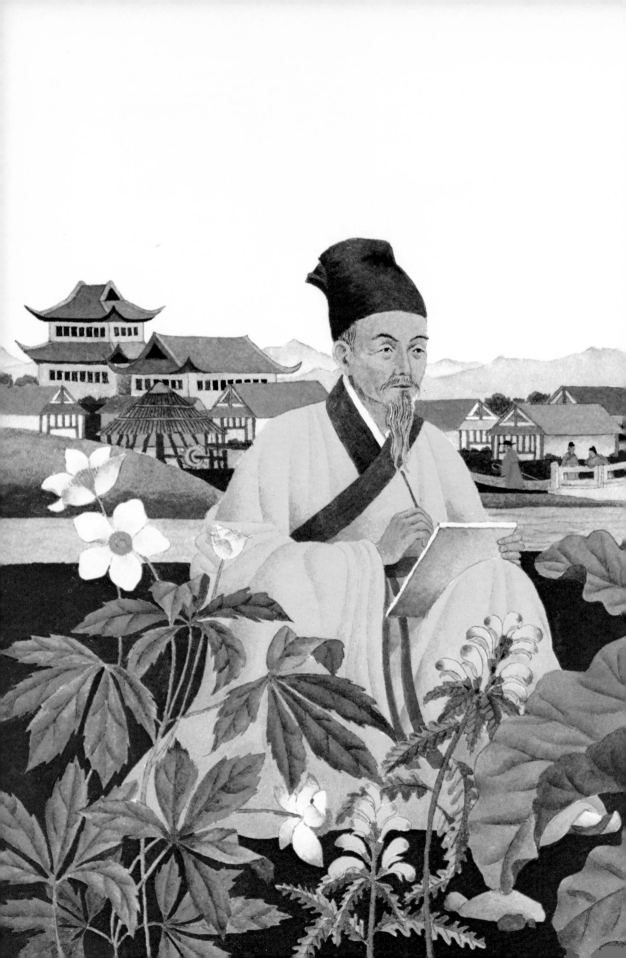

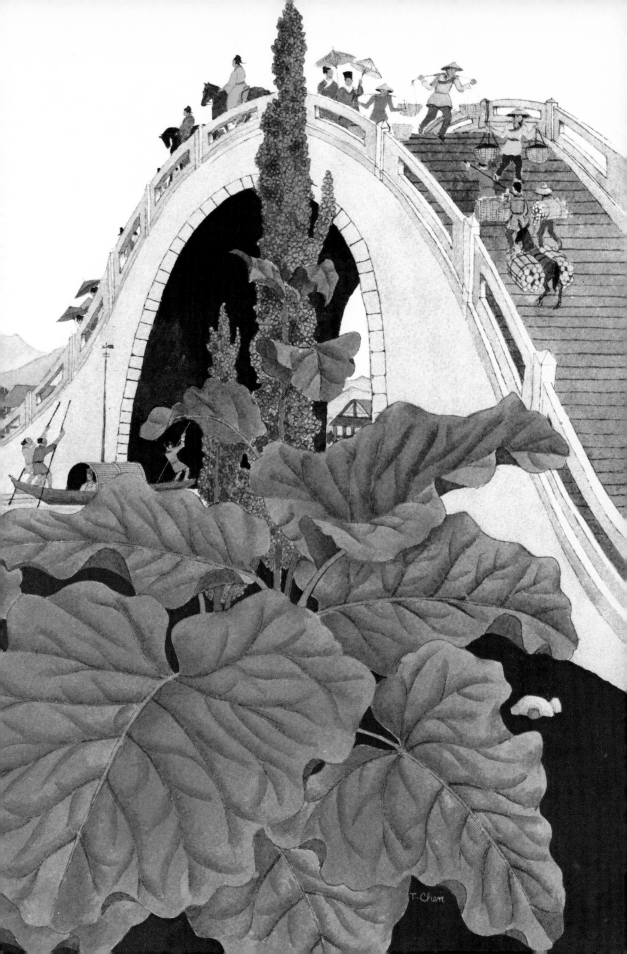

Sword-shaped leaves of showy alpinia surround a Chinese woman and her grandchild near the mountain village of Kenting in southwestern Taiwan. She gathers the plant's berries for use as a stomach powder. Villagers harvest many wild herbs from these hills for sale to Japanese drug manufacturers. Below, Lee Wu-lee, 78, Kenting's leading herbalist, doses her ailing water buffalo with a tonic made from ten different plants.

BOTH BY NATHAN BENN

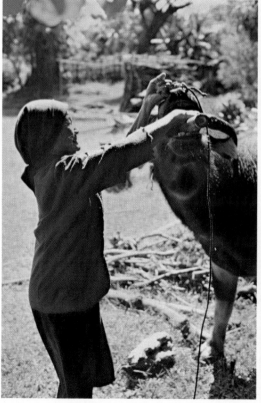

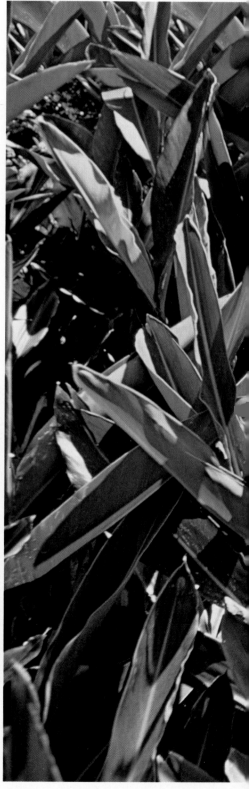

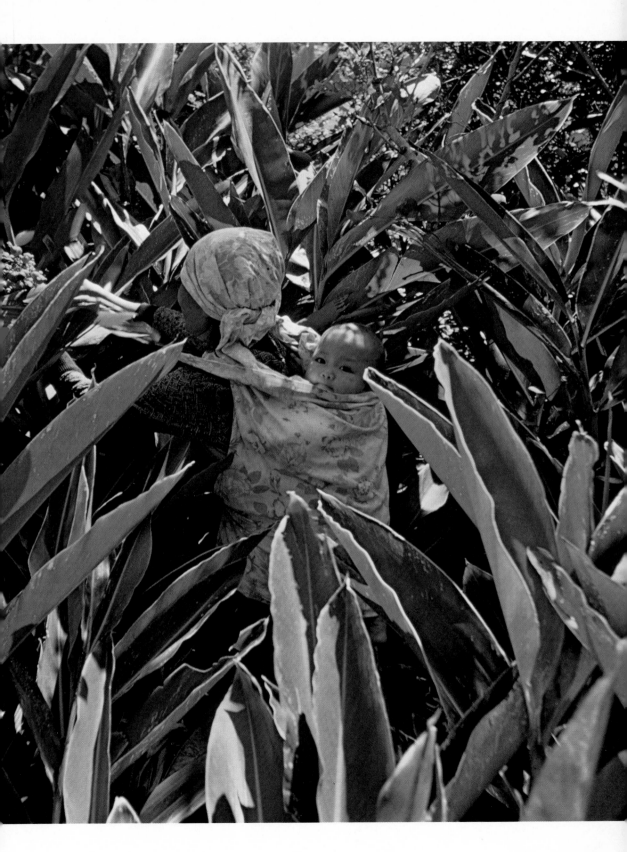

*Displaying stems of tasselflower — a fever depressant — pharmacy professor
Kan Woei-song lectures a class from the China Medical College during a
field trip to the herb-rich mountains of eastern Taiwan. A student
(far right) leaps to pick a leaf from a tree. During the course on medicinal
plants, the students make several such excursions to gather specimens.
They identify and study them using a textbook (right), which lists
nearly two thousand species. Formal medical education on Taiwan
combines ancient herbal techniques and modern clinical practices.*

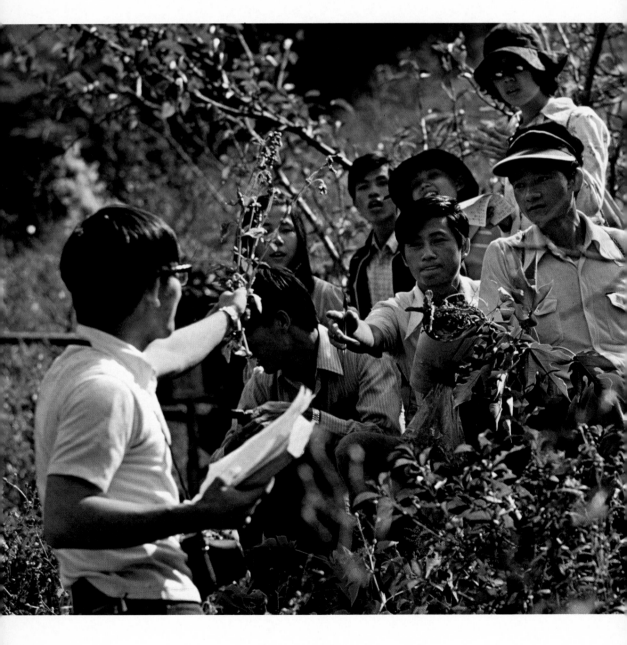

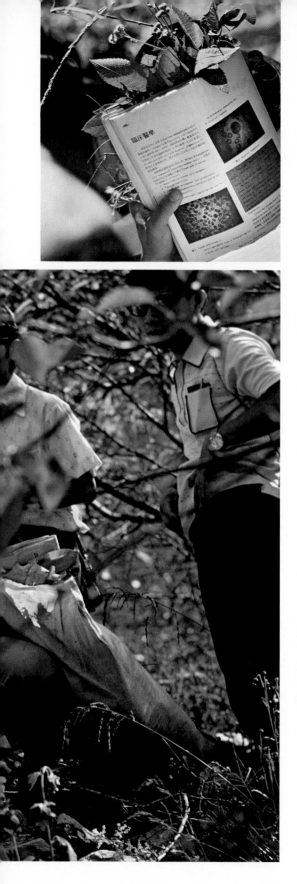

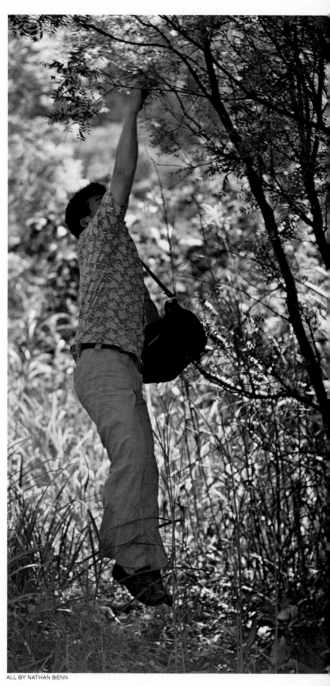

ALL BY NATHAN BENN

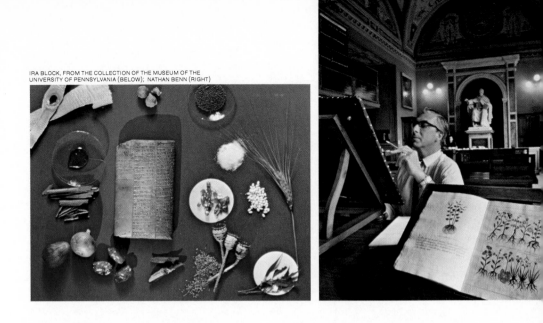

IRA BLOCK, FROM THE COLLECTION OF THE MUSEUM OF THE
UNIVERSITY OF PENNSYLVANIA (BELOW); NATHAN BENN (RIGHT)

raise mental and physical capacity for work. A combination of these factors can, perhaps, even lengthen life. More specifically, according to reports published by the Soviet Academy of Sciences, the use of ginseng drugs in experimental studies with animals has given encouraging results in cases of diabetes, neurosis, and radiation sickness.

In the United States, the medical profession has been slow to credit ginseng with anything but psychological benefits. Yet here, too, its demulcent, or soothing, effect on conditions such as gastrointestinal irritation is now recognized.

One American physician, the late Dr. Arthur R. Harding of Columbus, Ohio, anticipated most Western proponents of ginseng by many years. Dr. Harding gave up his general practice in the early 1900's to devote his life to cultivating the plant and experimenting with it on his patients. In his book, *Ginseng and Other Medicinal Plants,* written in 1908 and revised in 1972, he observed that ginseng root medication had "cured every case where I have used it with one exception and that was a case of consumption in its last stages. . . ."

But the Chinese still hold first place not only in the number of ginseng remedies, but also in herbal treatment as a way of life. Both the People's Republic of China—population more than 800 million—and the Republic of China on the island of Taiwan—population 16 million—carry on traditional and modern medicine side-by-side. In Taiwan, at least 6,000 pharmacies sell herbs and other natural products, and some 3,000 licensed traditional doctors write prescriptions for them.

Mainland China, however, is giving its people the biggest dose of herbs ever administered anywhere. Previously, a few trained physicians and public health groups had attempted to provide needed medical care in rural areas. Though these efforts met with modest success, political tur-

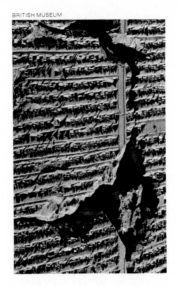

Documents from ancient civilizations record herbal remedies. Myrtle, thyme, barley, and other plants native to Mesopotamia encircle a 4,000-year-old Sumerian clay tablet (far left) listing prescriptions of natural products. The Aztec Herbal (left) rests in a library at the Vatican in Rome for a scholar's inspection. The Spanish had Aztec students compile this catalog of botanical remedies in 1522. The cuneiform tablet at right, one of 660 medical relics from the Assyrian Empire, dates from the 7th century B.C. It tells of medicinal plants and their uses.

moil through the 1940's and '50's hampered their development until the Communist Party Chairman, the late Mao Tse-tung, launched his own medical revolution in 1965.

Mao's extensive "red-and-rural" campaign required professionally equipped physicians from big-city hospitals to go among the people in mobile units, to share their lives, and to train local health workers—called barefoot doctors—in treating common ailments.

The result has been to create an army of paramedics, chosen for political and social dedication, who now number more than a million. In caring for the sick in communes all over the country, these barefoot doctors practice simple Western, as well as traditional Chinese, medicine. But their remedies are based mostly on herbs that often grow close by in fields and forests. Collected or cultivated, they are made into drug compounds in local factories.

"In Peking Province, one handbook carried by barefoot doctors contains 750 different herbal prescriptions for various diseases," said Dr. Norman Farnsworth after his recent visit to China. "Traditional Chinese medicine," he summed up, "is about 85 percent natural products, and about 15 percent acupuncture. Moreover, herbs are frequently applied as part of the acupuncture treatment."

As Sir William Osler, a Canadian-American physician and historian observed, "The desire to take medicine is perhaps the greatest feature which distinguishes man from animals."

Certainly the quest for the right prescription in the right amount has never been easy. In the beginning, most primitive peoples explained the mysteries of illness and injury as punishment for their sins or as the malevolence of some angry god. Thus the herbal and animal products in ancient remedies were often mixed by priests or temple physicians and given to patients with ceremonial incantations and prayers to divinities believed to control the destinies of ordinary mortals.

As experiments continued century by century, shrewd laymen as well as professional healers learned the hard way which plants were usually harmless and which innocent-looking ones carried death in their fruits and roots. So, gradually, each developing civilization accumulated its own science of cures, which was often fanciful or dangerous, but sometimes surprisingly effective.

How do we know this? The most direct and accurate knowledge that medical historians cite comes from a dozen or so original documents and other artifacts that still exist in tangible form.

Not long ago, I held in my hand a small clay tablet that is one of those precious objects. A collection of the world's oldest preserved prescriptions, it was inscribed in cuneiform characters 4,000 years ago by a pioneering physician of the Sumerian empire in what is now southern Iraq. I saw it at the Museum of the University of Pennsylvania in Philadelphia, where it is displayed as the major find of one of the University's expeditions to the excavated Sumerian city of Nippur.

I gazed at the strange, wedge-shaped symbols scratched into a broken bit of clay, and wondered what secrets they told. Fortunately, I met that day the most erudite interpreter possible, Dr. Miguel Civil. A cuneiform scholar with the Oriental Institute of Chicago, he has made the definitive translation of the 15 Sumerian prescriptions.

Most of the ingredients were collected from the vegetable kingdom, he told me. Some came from trees—myrtle, pear, fig, and myrrh—while others were native herbs such as thyme and mustard. The Sumerians also made medicines with animal products—bird and bat droppings, sheep's wool, powdered snakeskins, and hair balls from a cow's stomach. They mixed these medicines in solutions of water, wine, milk, and beer. They even added salt and saltpeter, having extracted and processed these substances in a manner that indicated at least a crude understanding of chemical reactions.

"But the most interesting aspect of the Sumerian tablet to me," Dr. Civil concluded, "was its rational approach to coping with illness without calling on the magic spells and religious appeals that played so large a part in many early cures."

Another priceless artifact that reveals tantalizing glimpses into man's first efforts to understand his world and its ills is known as the Ebers Papyrus. A 66-foot-long scroll written in Egyptian hieratic script 35 centuries ago, this durable record contains more than 800 medical recipes, intermingled with incantations and spells. It is considered Egypt's greatest medical document. Yet it came to light only in 1872, when Georg Ebers, the German Egyptologist for whom it was named, bought it from a collector of antiquities at Luxor.

Since then, Dr. Ebers' papyrus, displayed in the library of the Karl Marx University in Leipzig, Germany, has offered students of primitive medicine a rich source of information.

Some now feel that less attention should be paid to the superstitions and ritual surrounding the prescriptions, and more credit given to the genius of the assemblers of medications that bear a remarkably close resemblance to modern ones.

The Egyptians, for instance, prescribed castor oil as a laxative and as a scalp rub to make hair grow and shine. They prepared an extract of pomegranate root to expel intestinal worms; they made antiseptics of copper and other metallic salts for eye infections, and treated heart trouble with juice of the Mediterranean sea onion, one of the strongest heart stimulants known.

One Egyptian medication designed to quiet a restless child directs the healer to ". . . take pods of the poppy plant and add fly dirt that is on the wall. . . ." The opium content of this mixture was a startling precursor of today's modified paregoric that pediatricians frequently prescribe for colicky babies.

Roasted ox liver, a once-unlikely substance that the Egyptians swallowed to improve night vision, sounds perfectly reasonable now that we know about vitamin A's beneficial effect on eyesight. And the people of the Nile put moldy bread on wounds or took it internally for other ills millennia before scientists made penicillin and other antibiotics from mold cultures and soil bacteria.

As with the Egyptians, increasing information on the customs of the Babylonians and Assyrians leads historians to believe that rational medicine was carried on by these ancient peoples quite independently of their arts of exorcism and religious ceremonies of healing.

A big boost to the practical side came with the publication in 1923 of R. Campbell Thompson's translation of more than a hundred cuneiform tablets excavated at Nineveh from the buried library of King Ashurbanipal of Assyria, who reigned from 668 to 626 B.C. On these clay fragments, preserved at the British Museum in London, Dr. Thompson found symbols representing 250 plants, along with mineral and animal substances that went into Assyrian remedies. Many of the herbs they used were simples — garlic, licorice, and mustard, for example — familiar to herbalists everywhere. Others — deadly nightshade or belladonna, henbane, and thorn apple — must often have been lethal in those days, though we know now that they contain atropine, hyoscyamine, and scopolamine, prescribed by doctors to relax eye muscles and to relieve spasms.

Such curious links between ancient and modern medicine also surface in India's oldest existing literature, the *Rig Veda,* which dates to 1500 B.C. In its main medical text — the *Atharva Veda,* compiled about 700 B.C. — herbs and pure water are mentioned as therapeutic, and water was especially praised.

Still, a primitive people who knew nothing of the functions of their bodies could hardly be expected to find a scientific relationship between disease and treatment, cause and cure. So *Atharva Veda* "medicine" was made up largely of hymns to the gods for relief. Its herbs were picked by what came to be called the Doctrine of Signatures — a theory that diseases could be cured by plants or other objects resembling the affliction in color or shape. The *Atharva Veda,* for instance, makes much of the power of the lotus root to treat jaundice because of its yellow color.

It was not until the flowering of Greek civilization — when a respect for science and reason and a concern for the individual developed — that rational medicine, as we think of it, had its true beginnings.

Hippocrates, who lived from about 460 to 377 B.C., is best remembered for his oath outlining the moral responsibilities of all who enter the medical profession. But even more important as a signpost to the future was his innovation of a system of clinical observation of patients. As a physician at the Temple of Aesculapius, a kind of health spa dedicated to the God of Medicine on the island of Kos, Hippocrates prescribed diet, baths, and exercise, as well as hundreds of medicinal plants; then he carefully noted their effect on his patients.

Among the plants he used was the white willow, a large drooping tree that is one of the most common and salubrious of nature's gifts. The cuneiform sign for the willow appears frequently in prescriptions on the 4,000-year-old Sumerian tablet from Nippur.

The Ebers Papyrus lists a liquid from the tree — probably from its bark or twigs — which was mixed with figs, frankincense, beer, and other things, and "boiled, strained, and taken for four days to cause the stomach to receive bread."

Again, willow appears in Dr. Thompson's translation of the Assyrian tablets. And the Bible makes many references to these trees as a source of comforting shade and water. Remembering Zion by the rivers of Babylon, writes the author of Psalm 137, "we wept . . . [and] hanged our harps upon the willow. . . ."

But the most pertinent observations on willow medication in classical times were made by Pedanius Dioscorides, a surgeon and pioneer botanist hired by the Roman Emperor Nero in the first century A.D. to travel with his troops.

Moving with the Roman army along the shore of the Mediterranean Sea, Dioscorides studied and collected thousands of plants and samples of mineral and animal products. From these he assembled his five-volume *De Universa Medicina;* this massive work was the authoritative source for physicians for the next 1,500 years.

Describing willow, he used its Latin name *Salix,* and pointed out the astringent qualities that have made it popular for so long: ". . . the iuice out of ye leaues & barck . . . doth help ye griefs of the eares," goes one prescription in a 17th-century English translation, "and the decoction of them is an excellent fomentation for ye Gout." For good measure, Dioscorides added that the bark "being burnt to ashes and steeped in vinegar takes away cornes and other risings in the feet. . . ."

The willow saga was just starting, however, with Dioscorides. Claudius Galen, another noted Greek physician of the following century — whose name lives on in the term "galenicals" for plant preparations — regarded willow-bark extract as helpful in cleansing and healing eyes that were inflamed or infected.

Other authorities continued to stress willow's value against ailments ranging from colds to asthma. In *The Herball* of John Gerard, a monumental compilation of Elizabethan plants first published in London in 1597, the "vertues" of its leaves and bark included the power "to stay the spitting of Bloud [when] boiled in wine and drunke."

So widespread, indeed, have been the uses of the willow tree that Dr. Wayland Hand, folk medicine specialist at the Center for the Study of Comparative Folklore and Mythology at the University of California at Los Angeles, has recorded nearly a hundred accounts of magical and medical customs involving it. Dr. Hand keeps such references in a unique card index that he started 30 years ago. One card on Louisiana folklore in the early 18th century tells of treating a fever by lying down on a heap of cool willow leaves. When the leaves became warm, it was believed, the fever had miraculously been transferred to them.

The modern era of willow can perhaps be dated from the late 1700's, when many doctors substituted a bitter decoction from its bark for the less available and more expensive cinchona bark, which was then the chief remedy for malarial fevers.

But the final acceptance of willow products in scientific circles took place not in the woods and fields, but in the laboratory. In 1827, a French chemist named Leroux extracted the active substance in its bark that gave relief from pain. He named it "salicin," for the willow genus *Salix*.

Other scientists developed related compounds, but it was not until the 1890's that Felix Hofmann, a chemist with Friedrich Bayer and Company near Cologne, Germany, launched a successful career for one of them — acetylsalicylic acid — with the hope of finding a drug to help his arthritic father. As finally marketed in 1899, the new product was baptized with the more pronounceable name of aspirin. Later, the drug was moved completely into the laboratory, when its makers shifted from natural to synthetic sources. Eventually, aspirin would become the world's best-known medication.

Yet willow itself remains one of the historic drug plants whose example has led medical scientists to uncover the secrets of nature that form the basis of all modern remedies. And this process had begun nearly a century before aspirin came on the market with the achievement of a 20-year-old apothecary's assistant in Paderborn, a small German town.

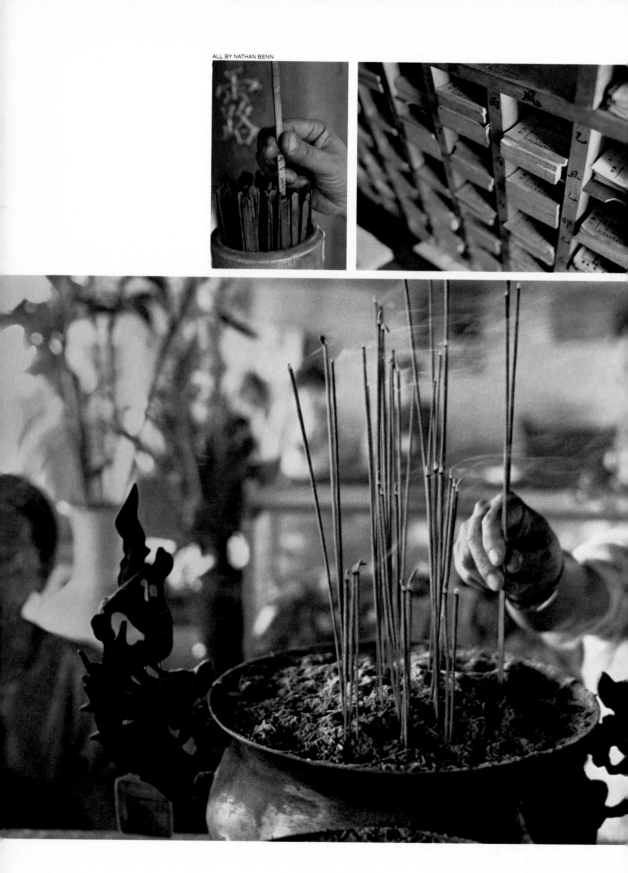

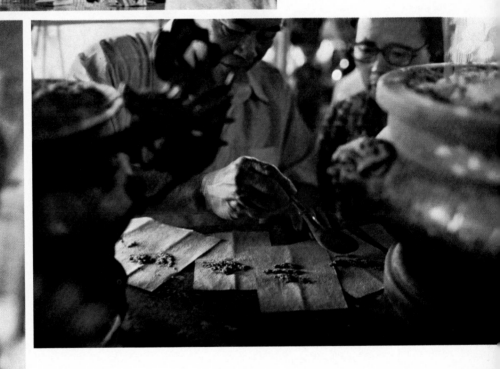

*Faith and herbal medicine converge at a Taoist
temple in Taiwan. A worshiper (left) burns herb-
covered incense sticks in a brass urn; after wrapping
the ash (above), he will carry it with him for luck and
good health. As part of a ritual, a woman (top, left)
selects one of sixty bamboo sticks. Each stick has
a corresponding prescription kept in a cabinet
with pigeonholes; she receives the prescription
for a botanical medication from an attendant.*

Age-old Oriental practices which treat internal ailments by stimulating certain points of the body continue at hospitals in Taiwan. Below, a doctor tests a man's arms following acupuncture for arthritis. Needles pierce the brow of a patient suffering from severe headaches as he times his treatment; another receives electrical acupuncture after a back operation. At right, a woman with a foot injury undergoes moxibustion—warming the skin with herbs smoldering inside a capsule.

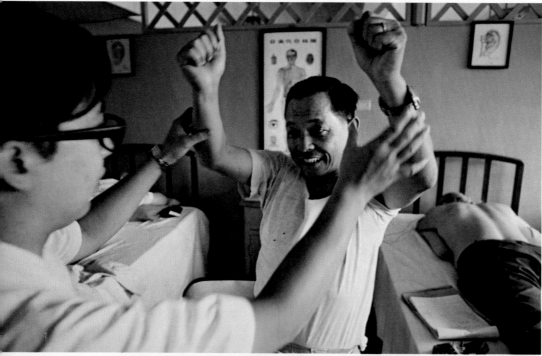

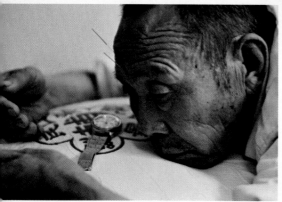

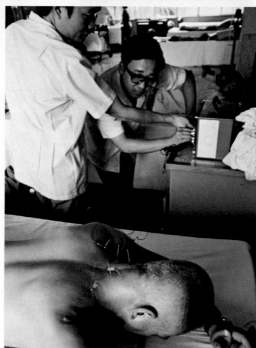

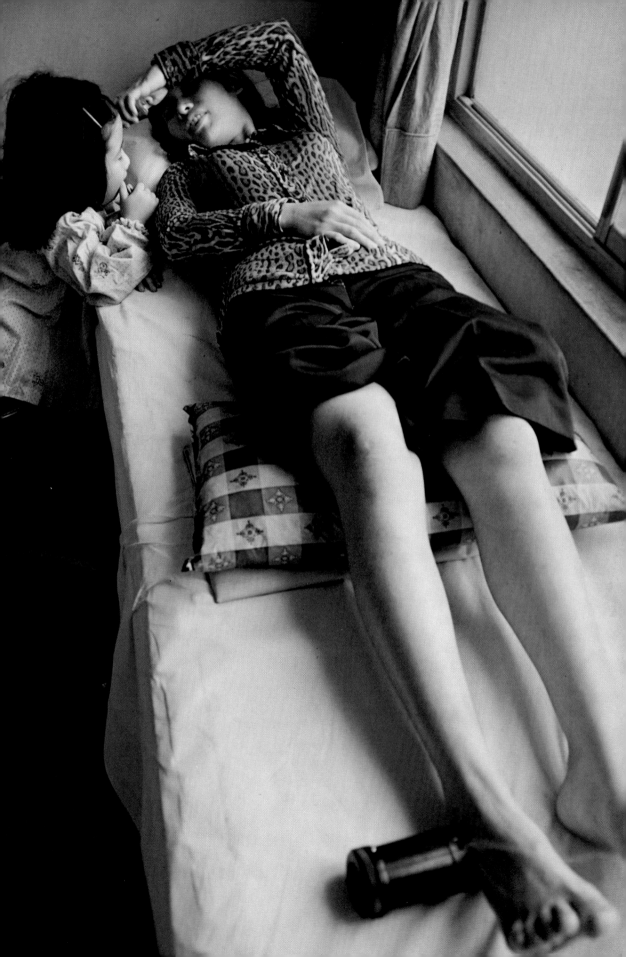

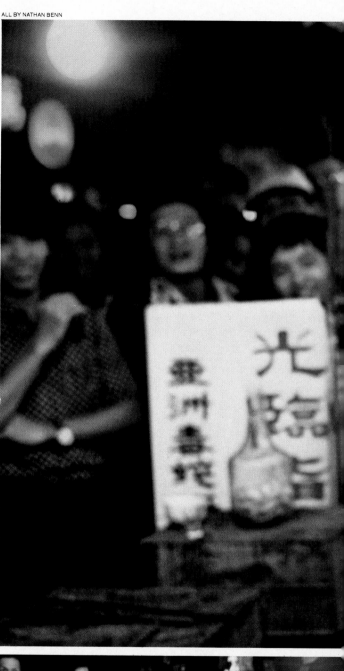

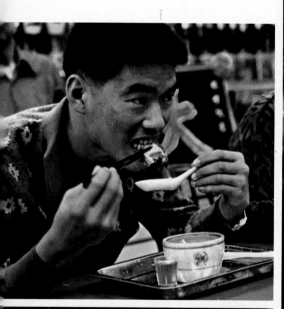

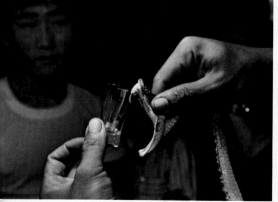

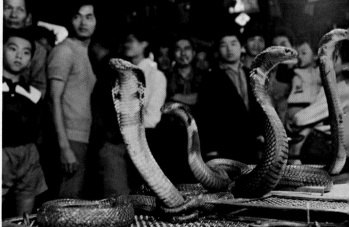

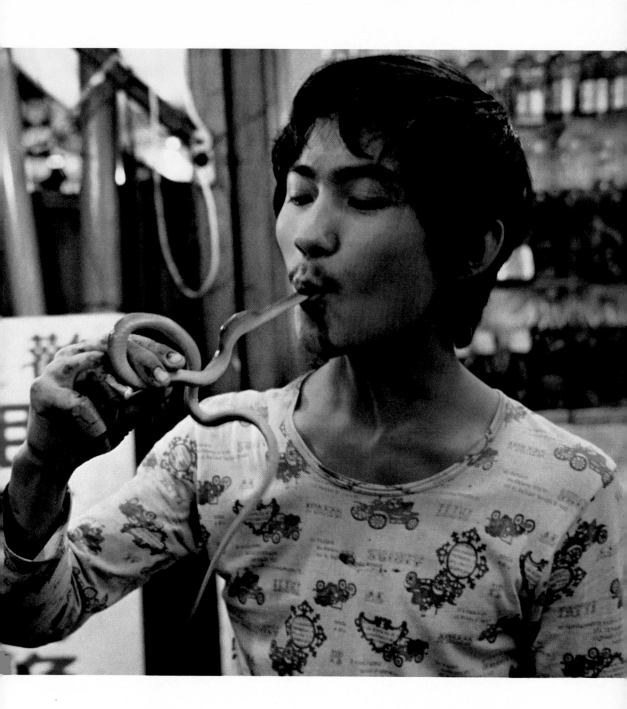

Luring buyers from competing snake shops in Yuan Huan, a market area in Taipei, Taiwan, a clerk handles a poisonous green snake. At left, cobras sway on top of their cages. Such shops—popular with the Chinese—offer snake medicines made from blood, venom, gall, and skin, and used to improve vision and to treat skin infections. At far left, a handler milks venom from a bamboo viper. A customer eats a thin soup containing snake meat.

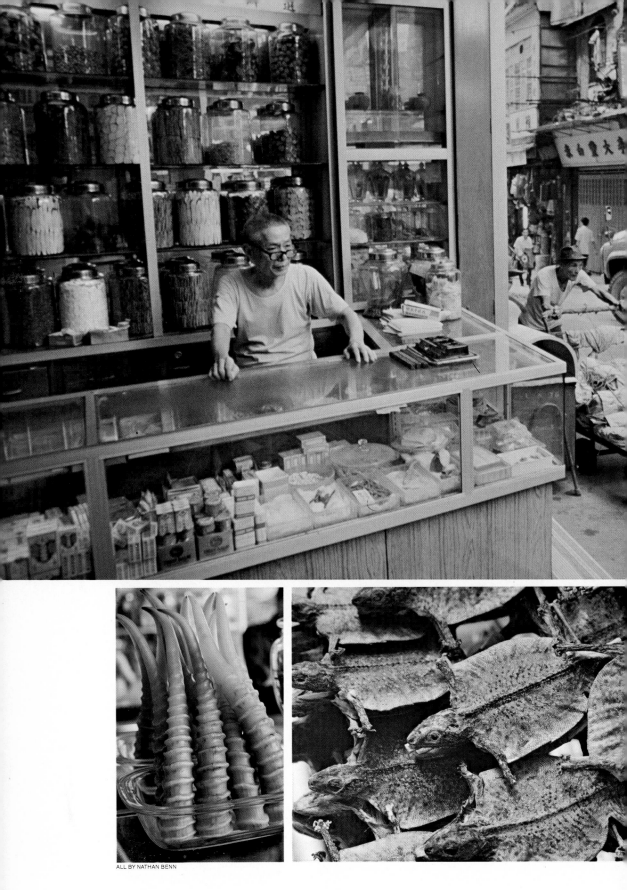

ALL BY NATHAN BENN

88

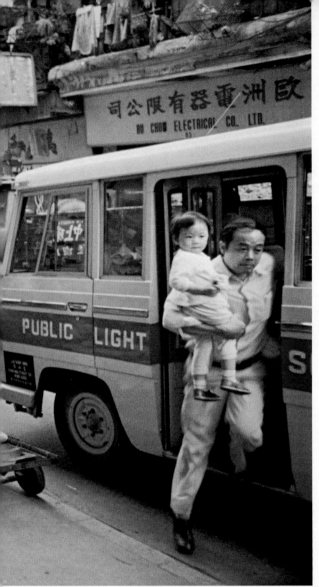

Ancient remedies fill the shelves of an apothecary shop in Hong Kong. Traditional offerings (below, left to right) include antelope horns, used in treating convulsions; geckos, used to combat asthma; sea dragon tails, an aphrodisiac; and a toad, whose skin, dried and powdered, may relieve heart trouble.

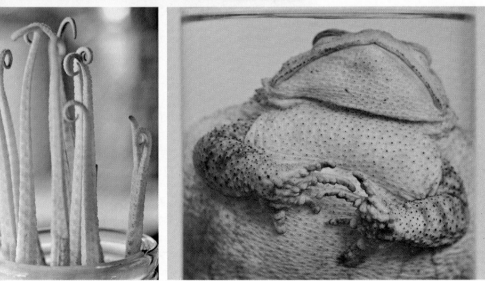

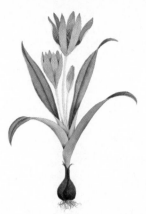

Dawn of Modern Medicine

HIS NAME was Friedrich Wilhelm Adam Ferdinand Sertürner—a rather grandiose cognomen for a young assistant pharmacist whose chemical competence was still unknown. But Sertürner had an idea that would change the course of medical history.

About 1803, he began experiments in his spare time in the back room of the Hof Apotheke, a pharmacy in Paderborn. His equipment was that of the ordinary apothecary shop of the time; his material was eight ounces of dry opium from the head of the poppy *Papaver somniferum;* his goal was to isolate from the plant the sleep-inducing factor whose good and evil influence had been known for centuries.

William Shakespeare had written of the poppy's "drowsy syrups" in *Othello,* and Thomas de Quincey, Sertürner's contemporary, would refer to his desperate addiction in *Confessions of an English Opium Eater* as the "abyss of enjoyment."

Sertürner soon succeeded in releasing opium's two-faced genie. He demonstrated the narcotic effects of the crystalline substance in tests on a mouse, four dogs, and four young men, including himself. He named his discovery "morphine" for Morpheus, the god of dreams in classical

Native doctor Mohamed Kifaru waits for patients seeking his herbal medication near Mtopanga, Kenya. In practice for some 30 years, he also teaches student herbalists methods and cures used for generations.

AUTUMN CROCUS (ABOVE)

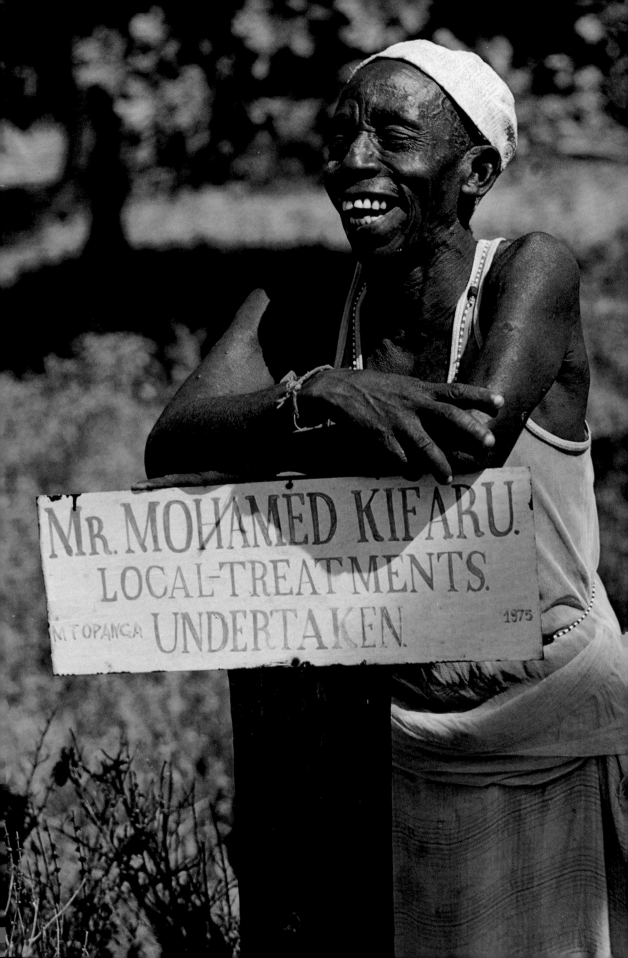

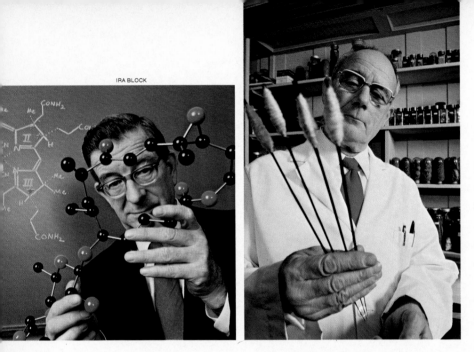

Scientists unlock the secrets of natural cures. Harvard chemist R. B. Woodward (far left), peers through the molecular model of an antibiotic. His work in synthesizing natural drugs won him a Nobel Prize in 1965. "Dean of the plant hunters," Harvard botanist Richard E. Schultes (left) holds

mythology. No other drug would ever earn more gratitude from patients and doctors for controlling pain. Of even greater value to the practice of medicine was Sertürner's discovery that morphine is an alkaloid. He thus laid the cornerstone of alkaloidal chemistry, which would make it possible in time to prescribe a precise dose for a specific disease.

As other chemists followed in Sertürner's footsteps, they extracted more plant alkaloids to form active bases for new medicines, many of which would alleviate, and sometimes cure, old ailments. Among the best known of these early discoveries were: emetine, still one of the most widely prescribed drugs for amoebic dysentery, extracted from the Brazilian ipecac root in 1817; strychnine, a powerful stimulant to the central nervous system, isolated from seeds of the *Strychnos nux-vomica* tree in 1818; quinine, the great malaria fighter, obtained from the bark of the South American cinchona tree in 1820; and cocaine, taken from the leaves of the Andean coca bush in 1860.

Other inquiring chemists discovered and added to the list of alkaloids more groups of biologically effective substances. These included glycosides, which come mainly from plants, and contain one or more sugars; hormones, which are natural secretions of plants and animals that stimulate the functions of glands and organs; and antibiotics, which are developed from one microorganism to weaken or kill others.

Eventually, with the march of pharmaceutical knowledge, daring innovators learned not only to extract and improve such active components of natural products, but also to decipher their molecular structures and use them as blueprints for man-made chemicals.

One man stands out in the competitive field of synthetic drugs with the brilliance of a searchlight cutting through a dark night. That man is Robert Burns Woodward, professor of chemistry at Harvard University.

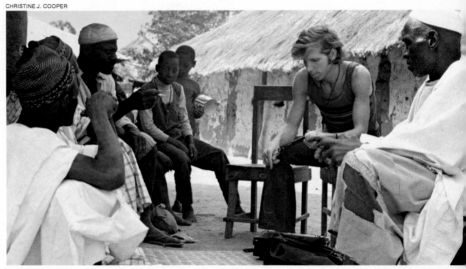

blowgun darts collected in the Amazon River Basin. From the deadly curare tipping the darts came a muscle-relaxant drug. Anthropologist Matt Schaffer interviews Mandinko elders in Senegal. With his wife, ethnobotanist Christine Cooper, he recorded their tribal history and medical traditions.

In 1965, he won the Nobel Prize for establishing the nature of the active constituent in many medicinal plants, and for creating in his laboratory other chemical structures of valuable synthetic medicines.

When I visited Dr. Woodward — a handsome man with dark blue eyes — in his blackboard-lined office at Harvard, I asked how he and his collaborators around the world had been able to solve the inner mysteries of so many vital substances, such as quinine and quinidine, penicillin, cortisone, cholesterol, chlorophyll, and vitamin B_{12}.

My question, I realized, was a little like that of the physics student who telegraphed Albert Einstein for an explanation of his Theory of Relativity by return telegram. But Dr. Woodward managed to simplify the complexities of his work by skipping the diagrams and molecular patterns that usually fill his blackboard, and concentrating instead on medical aspects of his discoveries and the challenge of the search.

"Probably the most practical result of our work with quinine was finding out how to make quinidine from it," he said. "Quinidine occurs in nature in cinchona bark, but in much smaller quantities than quinine, which also comes from the bark. We developed a process for converting quinine into quinidine, and made readily available a medicine that is used quite extensively, especially for people who have atrial fibrillation — palpitations of the heart.

"Penicillin was the first of a large class of antibiotics to be isolated," he continued. "That was soon after the outbreak of World War II, and it led to a huge Anglo-American program to determine its structure, and later to synthesize it. I directed part of that program, and ended up discovering the correct penicillin structure," he said.

Dr. Woodward spoke of many other drugs whose life secrets he has plumbed, including tetracycline — like penicillin, a mold antibiotic — which

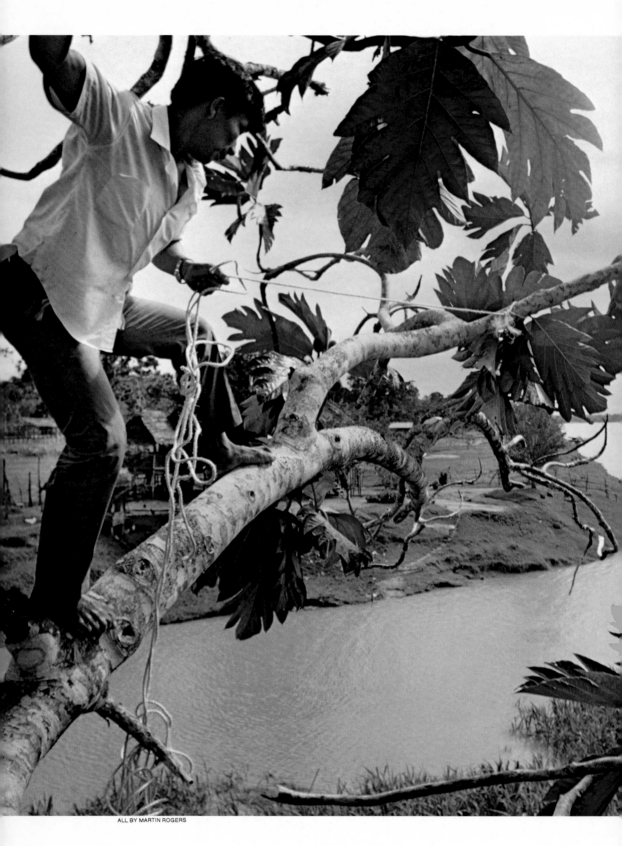

94

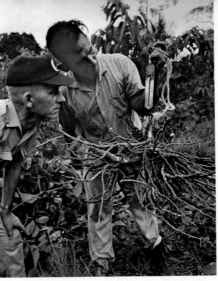

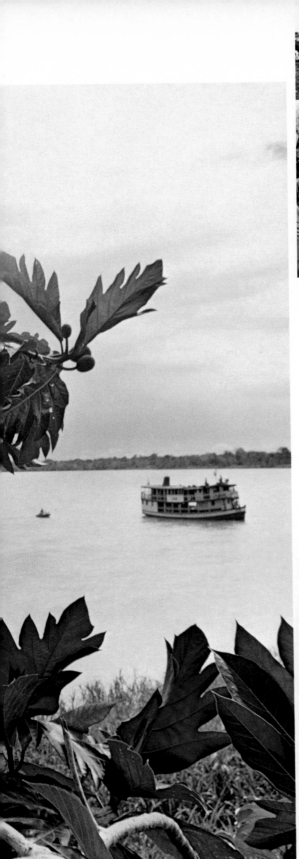

Along the Amazon River, a crewman gathers breadfruit to take to the Frannewood III. *The vessel provided drying facilities and living quarters during a six-year project sponsored by the Amazon Natural Drug Company to find new drugs from plants. Assistants (below) prepare some of the hundreds of plants collected. On shore, (above) workers weigh freshly dug roots.*

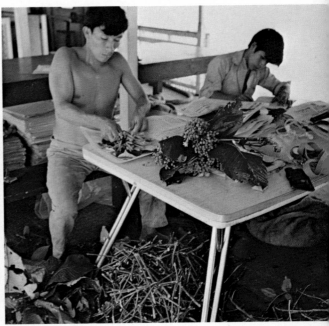

he synthesized after demonstrating its natural structure. "Another successful discovery was the hormone cortisone and its related compounds. They've had widespread medical use in the treatment of rheumatoid arthritis and as general anti-inflammatory agents."

After several hours of talking with Dr. Woodward about his work, I asked him one final question. Why has he taken on the enormously difficult problem of analyzing nature's chemical structures and putting together new ones? He pondered his answer, then began, "It's partly because of the detective work involved—the satisfaction of solving a puzzle. There's an attraction, too, in the day-to-day operations, an almost sensuous pleasure in the beauty of the colored substances and the orderly patterns of the crystals and molecules, as revealed when you pass X rays through them. This method of determining the structure of a substance is now immensely facilitated by the computers that do the complicated arithmetic for us.

"It's also a fantastic challenge. Sometimes I can more or less follow the processes that nature evolved through billions of years. At other times I have to make up my own plans and procedures as I go along. The paths to follow are infinite.

"But always," he added thoughtfully, "it's long, hard work. Vitamin B_{12}, a substance indispensable in treating pernicious anemia, took 13 years to synthesize, and was the result of collaboration between myself and Professor Albert Eschenmoser of the Swiss Federal Institute of Technology, with the help of a hundred other colleagues."

Although synthetic vitamin B_{12}, which was produced in 1972, has not come into medical use because of the availability of the natural substance, scientists in the field say that this fact is less important than the knowledge of new chemical principles revealed by the work. Beyond the practical benefits of the achievement itself lies the promise of developing more effective medicines.

Most people are aware, of course, that chemists play a necessary role in getting raw materials to the assembly lines of manufacturers who turn out the pills and salves, lotions and potions for the pharmaceutical market. Less well known are the many other professions involved in the eternal quest for new and better medicines.

Specialists in these fields range from plant hunters in the wild to big-city physicians; from biologists testing the activity of microorganisms to archeologists digging for evidence of ancient drug use. In fact, as I talked with many of the talented men and women in these varied disciplines, I came to feel that they form a kind of club whose members meet from time to time in national and international symposiums to pool the results of their latest investigations and discoveries.

Dr. Richard Evans Schultes, director of the Botanical Museum at Harvard University, combines at least three of the disciplines—plant hunter, ethnobotanist, and professor of natural sciences.

Near the beginning of his 40-year career in field and academic work, he spent a long exploratory period, from 1941 to 1954, paddling the streams and slogging through the jungles of South America's Amazon River Basin. Along the way, he suffered malaria and beriberi. But this professor, I learned after climbing the stairs to his fourth-floor eyrie in the Botanical Museum, is more concerned with results than with such hazards. He considers them part of his job.

In his clipped Bostonian accent, he stressed the value of plants in developing other cures and recalled the exploits of his boyhood hero, Richard Spruce—a 19th-century British botanist whose explorations and discoveries in the Amazon lured Dr. Schultes along the same paths. Not only was Spruce one of the great pioneers of botanical history, Schultes said, but he also had a remarkable perception of the enormous wealth in the jungle waiting to be tapped. Despite the limitations of botanical knowledge in his day, Spruce estimated that the Amazon Basin contained perhaps 140,000 plant species.

Dr. Schultes, during his long visit to the region, gathered, pressed, and dried about 24,000 specimens of plants—many of them previously unknown—which he presented to the Harvard botanical collections. Among these, in addition to rare orchids and wild rubber, were various exotic narcotics. These are used as medicine and in religious and magical ceremonies by some of the world's most primitive tribes.

Penetrating the rain forests and tributaries of the great river, Schultes made friends with the Indians and studied their ways of healing with nature's products. During one visit with the Yukunas of eastern Colombia, he was invited to join the tribe—an honor he ranks as high as any of his scientific and governmental awards. In 1970, he revisited his Yukuna friends, and took along his ten-year-old son, Evans, to enjoy the reunion.

Since 1954, when Schultes returned to the United States and resumed an academic career at Harvard, he has gone back to the Amazon every year except one. So far, these trips have brought the university's herbariums 6,000 additional plants for further identification and possible chemical and clinical study.

In early 1977, Schultes headed a major international expedition into the western part of the Amazon Basin. Its members included Dr. Timothy Plowman—a former student—and ten scientists from Sweden, Switzerland, England, Peru, and Colombia. The group assembled at the mouth of the Caraparaná River and headed upstream aboard the *Alpha Helix,* a research ship provided by the Scripps Institution of Oceanography in La Jolla, California.

"Some of us collected on land and brought back the plants for others to

Overleaf: Friedrich Sertürner notes the effects of morphine on a mouse. In 1803—in a medical breakthrough—the German pharmacist isolated the plant alkaloid morphine, the opium poppy's painkilling substance.

97

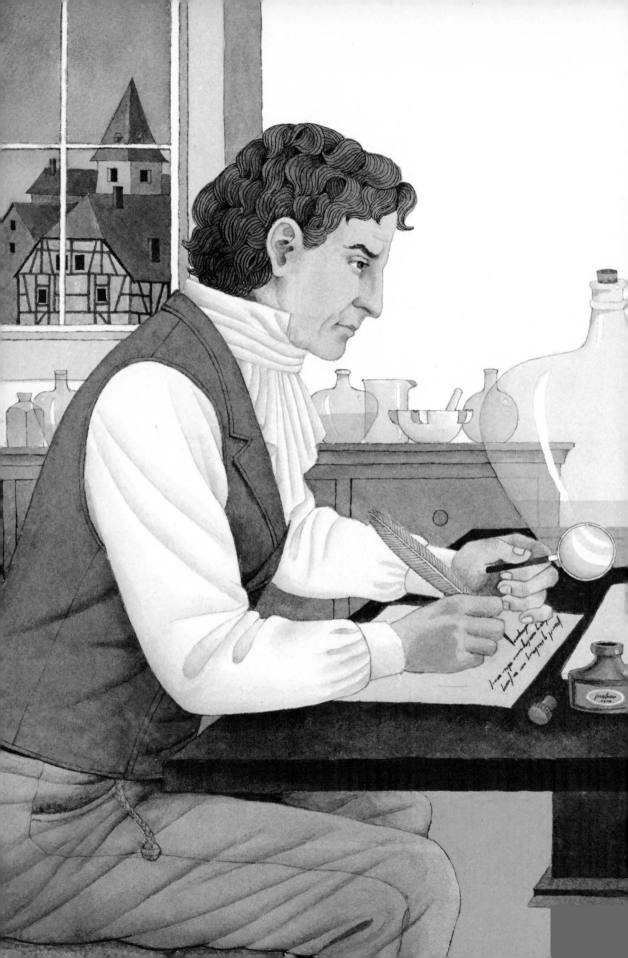

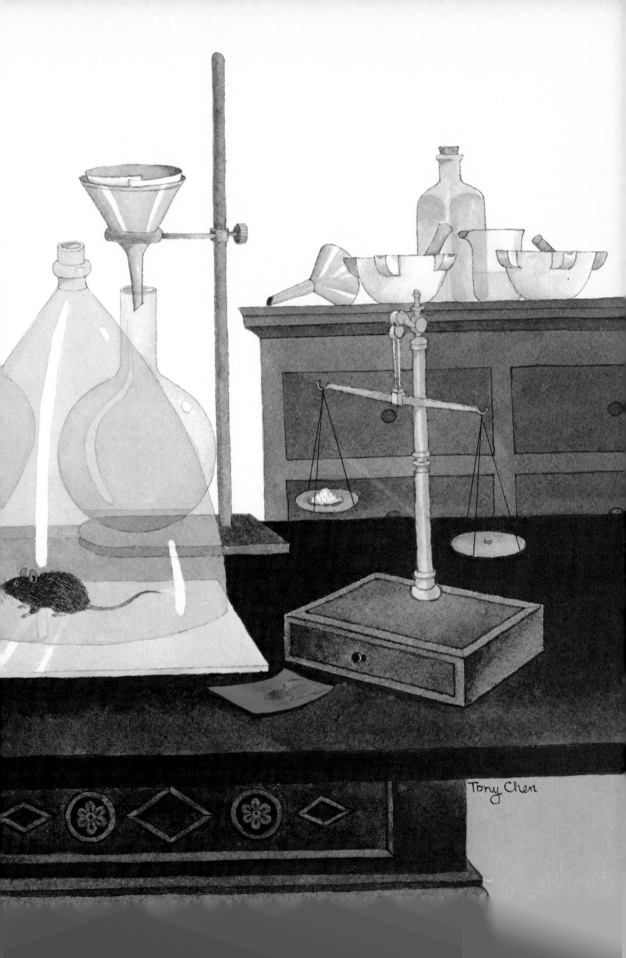

screen in the ship's excellently equipped laboratories," Dr. Schultes explained. "Our general objective was to investigate hallucinogenic, poisonous, and medicinal constituents of the area's plants, and the only way to do it effectively was to gather living material and analyze it on the spot.

"To be more specific," he said, "one of our main subjects was the coca plant, whose leaves are swallowed by the Indians of the Amazon in powdered form, and chewed whole by the peoples of the high Andes. Tim Plowman was especially concerned with the coca plant, having just completed a three-year field study on the mountain species. His aim in the lowlands was to pinpoint the differences, botanical and chemical, between the cocas of the two regions. This could be quite important. Most people dismiss coca chewing as a vice related to its cocaine content. However, the whole plant is not only nonaddictive, but, as Plowman has already reported, is also richer in vitamins and minerals than are dozens of South American food plants."

Among other activities, Dr. Schultes is compiling a book—his seventh—that will bring colleagues the results of field expeditions going back to his original 13-year collections in the Amazon. Published in loose-leaf form, this book will contain plant identifications, descriptions, and uses by native peoples of the area.

"I'll probably have five or six hundred plants cataloged, including notes on their medicinal and narcotic use," Schultes said. "If their chemistry has been analyzed, I'll include that information; but many have never been studied before. Lately I've concentrated on plants that the Indians use to treat such problems as skin fungus—common in the jungle—or 'pains in the chest' that could mean heart ailments. Who knows, maybe some remarkable new drug may come out of these rain forests."

Meantime, scientists on the trail of primitive medical folklore can turn to a remarkable book and follow leads culled from two and a half million field notes attached to plant specimens gathered for the collections of the Arnold Arboretum and Gray Herbarium at Harvard. This catalog of plants and places covers firsthand ethnographic details collected by botanists around the world. It was compiled by Dr. Siri von Reis Altschul, another of Schultes' students.

"The stories behind some of the collections are very interesting," said Dr. Altschul, a former fashion model. "Reading between the lines of many of these entries, you come to understand the difficult conditions under which collectors sometimes worked. And you almost feel their sudden pleasure in discovering an exotic species and learning how primitive peoples have used it."

After reading her book, entitled *Drugs and Foods from Little-Known Plants,* I, too, marveled at the courage and persistence of those knowledge seekers who climbed mountains and crossed deserts and rain forests in search of medicinal plants.

Year by year, such discoveries continue. Not long ago, I met a young ethnobotanist named Christine Cooper, who, with her anthropologist husband, Matt Schaffer, had just returned from field research with a West African tribe. Their studies may offer more clues to tomorrow's medicines. Supported by a Rhodes Scholarship and a National Geographic Society grant, the couple lived for 18 months among the Mandinko people in the Pakao region of Senegal. Using their respective professional skills, they recorded many facets of the tribe's religious and sociological history, along with details of their customs in treating diseases with local plants. It was not until their return to the United States that Christine and Matt learned of the Mandinkos' sudden fame as the ancestral tribe of Alex Haley, author of the best-selling book *Roots*.

"The Mandinkos are enormously fascinated by plants," Christine said. "My husband and I spent hundreds of hours in the woods with their botanical experts, who are usually game hunters or healers, and sometimes both. We helped them dig herbs and cut branches, leaves, and bark from various trees, and we were amazed at how quickly they found the ones they wanted.

"Although some Mandinkos have been Muslims for centuries, they still follow pre-Islamic practices and ceremonies using products of the trees that surround their village," Christine told me. "The most important of these trees is the *fara,* which they use for both magical and medicinal purposes. For its sacred role, they strip off the blood-red inner bark and make a costume for a terrifying figure called the *Kangkurao.* Behind his demon mask, the Kangkurao stalks about, clanking his machetes together and uttering inhuman shrieks—all part of his job to enforce order and scare workers into more enthusiasm for village tasks.

"As medicine, they consider extracts and lotions from parts of the fara tree especially good for malaria, eye diseases, and stomachaches. They also have a number of standard plant remedies, such as *pelinkumfo* for parasitic worms, and *katirao* for snakebite. Matt just missed having to test their snakebite treatments when spitting cobras twice came within a couple of inches of striking him."

These people bathe a lot, the couple learned, and apply many of their remedies in the form of washes made by steeping or boiling plant substances. The leaves of one bush with white, yellow, and violet flowers—a highly poisonous plant known to botanists as *Datura metel*—is a popular ingredient for various prescriptions. But Mandinkos never drink it or use it as a narcotic. They apply it to the body only as a wash or as a poultice for skin diseases, and particularly in cases of breast cancer. One woman healer told Christine that she had relieved the pain of many breast cancers with it, and even claimed to have cured some. Modern medical researchers do not scoff at such statements. Recent investigations into old folklore treatments for cancer have turned up a number of plants having tumor-resistant qualities—some of them closely related to *Datura metel.*

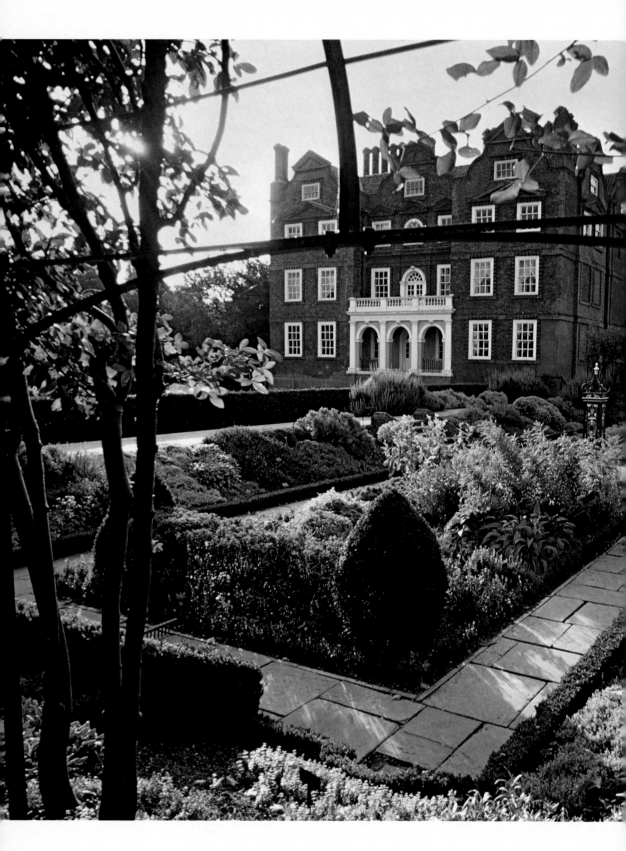

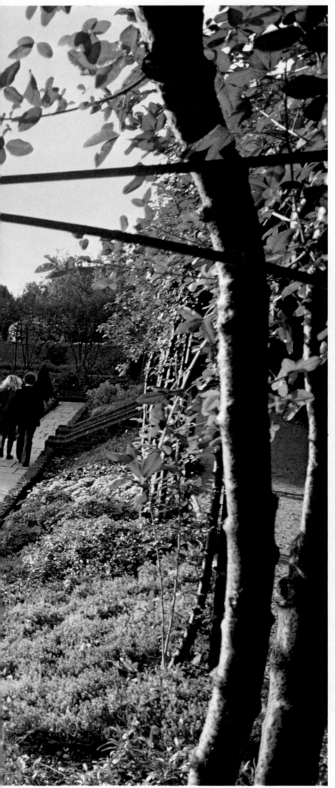

Herbs flourish in the 200-
year-old Royal Botanic
Gardens of Kew, England—
one of the world's major
centers for plant studies.
Gardener Philip Lusby waters
sage, an herb that "expelleth
winde, drieth the dropsie,
helpeth the palsie," claimed
a writer in the 1600's.

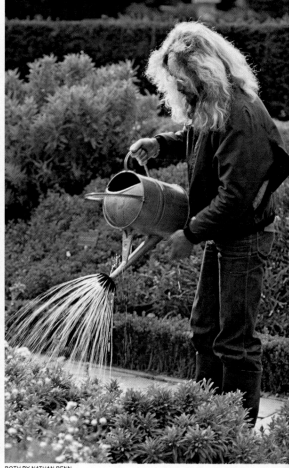

BOTH BY NATHAN BENN

In what we consider our more civilized world of mass-produced drugs, few consumers have any idea of where nature's raw ingredients come from, or how they reach the manufacturers.

To see how regional distributors collect wild plants in the United States, I traveled into the Appalachian hill country that provides the drug market with the major share of its domestic botanicals. In Boone, North Carolina, I visited the Wilcox Drug Company, largest and oldest of the area dealers. I hopped on one of their big trucks making a round of rural families who regularly dig, clip, and peel off such plant parts as witch hazel leaves, slippery elm bark, wild black cohosh and mayapple roots, and the curious lobelia herb — also called Indian tobacco — which is sold to help smokers break the habit.

The driver, Ralph Proffit, seemed to know everyone — including children, dogs, and cats — along bumpy roads winding past small mountain homes. Beeping the horn in advance, he stopped frequently, weighed the piled-up burlap bags filled with dried vegetation, wrote out checks to the gatherers, and drove on.

"We may make as many as 50 pickups a day," Ralph told me. "On a good day, I've hauled nearly nine tons."

Later, I saw some of the same Appalachian plants in warehouses at America's three leading manufacturing and import-export firms in botanicals — S. B. Penick, the Meer Corporation, and the Dr. Madis Laboratories. All are headquartered in New Jersey within a 20-mile radius. Each annually processes millions of pounds of plant products into tinctures and extracts for the pharmaceutical and other trades. These three companies send executives and scientists around the world to establish supply lines. They retain regional and local collectors, hire individual farmers, and sometimes raise their own crops where desired plants grow well.

When I visited their factory-laboratory compounds, I saw huge machines that clean and wash, grind and pulverize incoming materials; roller conveyors that move them about; and giant percolators using organic solvents and specialized equipment that process crude substances into extracts. I passed room-size spray driers that send atomized liquids over air heated to 400° F., and enormous blender tanks in which powders are finally mixed and standardized.

Each of the three companies has its own specialties. Penick, which started in the early 1900's as a small plant-collecting business, now has a large stake in chemicals, such as antibiotics and narcotics. Meer, which celebrated its 50th anniversary in 1976, specializes almost exclusively in large inventories of many kinds of botanicals, botanical extracts, and water-soluble gums. Madis Laboratories, established in Europe in 1942, emphasizes fast extractions with ultramodern equipment and highly automated procedures.

Now under way at Penick is a pioneering effort with the opium poppy. As Penick's vice president, William Thawley, explained it to me, the project developed after Turkey—the world's largest producer—banned all poppy cultivation under a 1971 agreement with the United States. This agreement was designed to curtail illicit diversion of raw material for the production of heroin.

Four years later, when it became clear that heroin traffic was still flourishing with opium allegedly smuggled from other countries, Turkey again permitted its farmers to grow poppies. They were not allowed, however, to return to the old practice of lancing the plant's unripe head, or capsule, and removing its gummy opium content. Instead, the government of Turkey buys the mature, dried capsules from the producers, and resells them as "poppy straw." To derive heroin from this material is a much more costly and complex operation. Penick chemically processes morphine, codeine, and other products from the poppy heads. It is the only company licensed by the Federal Government to do so.

Occasionally a dealer in botanicals has an opportunity to provide supplies of some promising plant believed to be of medicinal value because of old folklore usage or modern chemical findings. Such a plant was the Madagascar periwinkle, a handsome rose-and-white ornamental. In the 1950's it was found to contain alkaloids that indicated promise in fighting Hodgkin's disease and childhood leukemia. The investigating drug firm, Eli Lilly and Company of Indianapolis, asked the Meer Corporation to collect the initial laboratory specimens, and the hunt was on.

"This was the glamorous one in our gathering of plants for scientific investigation," said Dr. William Meer, the corporation's vice president and technical director. "It was also a tough one. We first had to identify the correct species, then arrange for its collection at the right season of the year, get it through the mails, and have its admittance approved by the Food and Drug Administration. We also had to set up sampling points in such potential producing areas as Madagascar, Australia, South America, South Africa, Europe, and India.

"Later, after further testing proved that the plant's beneficial substances were in its leaves, we furnished tons of this material for Lilly's first large-scale extractions—most of it from our own farm in southern India. Eventually, of course, clinical results demonstrated that the Madagascar periwinkle's alkaloids were, indeed, effective in bringing about high percentages of remissions in Hodgkin's disease and leukemia. And it was a great satisfaction to us here to have had a part in launching this successful program."

So we come from the wilderness to the laboratory and finally to the ailing patient for whom all these efforts are being made. But the story is not yet finished. After the patient takes the prescription, I wondered, how does the medicine travel through the body, and work on the area affected by the illness?

These are fundamental questions that hint at the mystery of life itself.

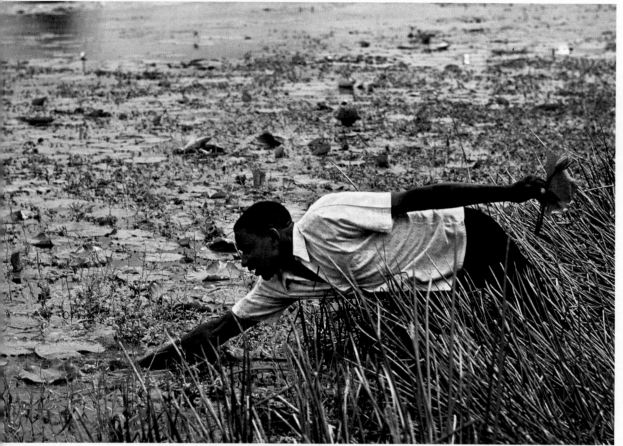

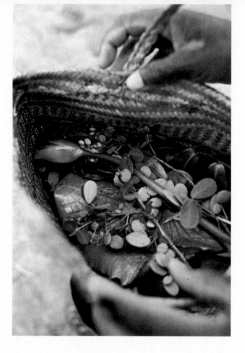

Plagued with bad dreams caused by "the devils of night," six-year-old Katana of Kenya receives treatment from his brother Kahindi Ngala. The healer rubs water-soaked leaves over the boy's body. Ngala, still in training at 28, learns medical traditions passed down through the centuries. Above, he picks water lily tubers, good for fevers, along Kenya's coast— an area noted for native doctors and curative herbs. A straw bag holds plants used to ease ailments ranging from worms to "fevers and devils."

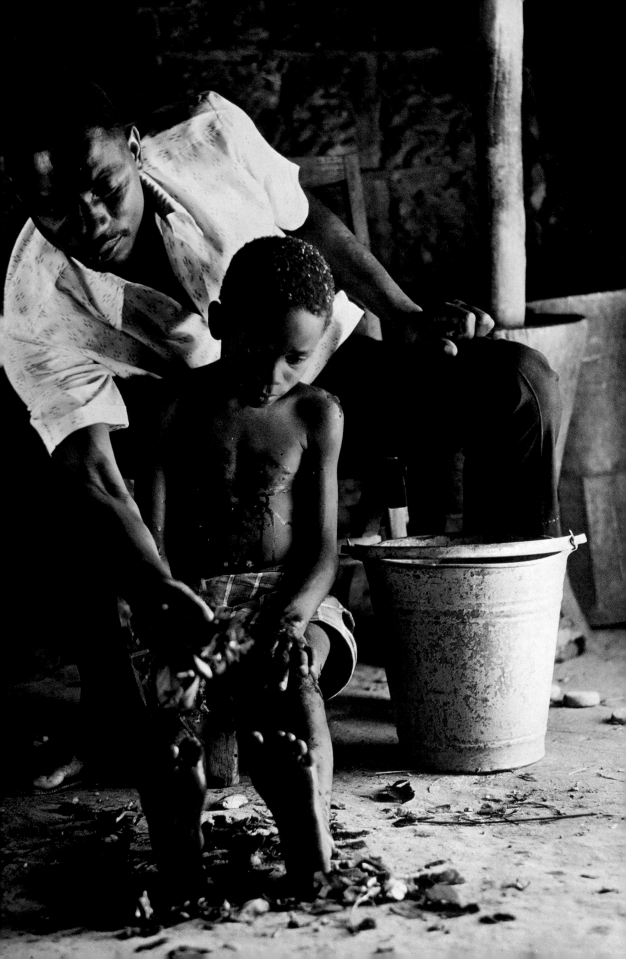

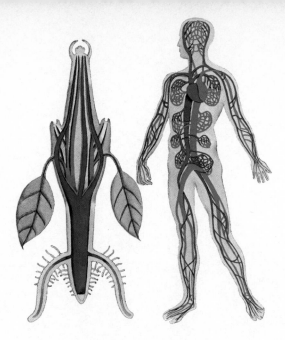

Living factories: Humans and plants, each formed of cells, have parallel systems for functions such as circulation, shown here in red and blue. The veins and arteries of a man work in the same way as a plant's stem passages to absorb, break down, and transport vital food and oxygen.

Every organism, whether animal or plant, is a living laboratory producing alkaloids, hormones, glycosides, and other chemical constituents according to its nature. Moreover, such organisms, including man, are made up of the same indestructible elements found in the universe — hydrogen, oxygen, carbon, nitrogen, calcium, and iron, plus small amounts of other minerals and chemicals. Despite this impressive range of elements, however, our total intrinsic value — chemically speaking — comes to only about $5 a person.

The actual mechanisms of drug action within the body have always offered one of the most fascinating — but least understood — areas of pharmaceutical investigation. The autumn crocus, a fall-blooming meadow saffron, provided researchers with the first inkling of drug action on human organisms. Its role in the treatment of gout reaches back more than two thousand years. But not until 1889 did scientists learn that colchicine, extracted from the crocus seed, stops cell division. As a result, it reduces inflammation and swelling, and thus removes the symptoms of gout. Just how it stops cell division and produces these pain-relieving effects unfortunately remains a mystery.

One of the first scientists to suggest that the answer might lie in the interaction of drugs with natural chemicals in the body's cells was Paul Ehrlich, pharmacologist and bacteriologist, who worked in Germany in the early 1900's. He was specifically trying to find a cure for syphilis that would destroy the disease-causing parasite without killing the patient along with it. On his 606th test, Ehrlich discovered an arsenic-containing compound that he called arsphenamine. It was later given the trade name Salvarsan. This drug was very crude; it took too long to work, and was so toxic that it was sometimes a toss-up whether the parasite or the patient would survive. But Ehrlich was successful in enough cases to make the result a great event — a forerunner of the modern antibiotics initiated with the discovery of penicillin by Alexander Fleming of England, who was later knighted for the achievement.

The son of a Scottish farmer, Fleming was working to find an agent against such infectious diseases as pneumonia and diphtheria, and his achievement was one of those happy accidents of medical history. At St. Mary's Hospital in London in 1928, he noted that a green mold on a culture plate was destroying staphylococcus bacteria. He named the mold *Penicillium*. During the next year, after testing the drug against many different kinds of bacteria, he reported, "Penicillin is non-toxic to animals in enormous doses and is non-irritant. . . . it may be an efficient antiseptic." For ten years a team of Oxford University scientists headed by Howard Florey investigated the therapeutic value of penicillin. Finally, with their first human case, a local bobby, the combined efforts gave medicine an antibiotic that destroyed the parasite without harming the cell.

With such an introduction, American scientists began searching for ways to grow the mold in quantity and at a reasonable cost. In the beginning they found that the mold grew best on the stems of decaying cantaloupes. They extracted this mold and placed it in a medium to multiply. During World War II, Yale University and the Mayo Clinic conducted the first clinical trials, and they were so successful that the drug almost immediately came into wide demand. However, there were no clues for more than a decade as to how penicillin interacted with the body's cells.

Then in 1975, John Hughes and Hans Kosterlitz, two doctors in Scotland engaged in research on drug addiction, discovered that morphine from the opium poppy acts on specific areas in the brain called receptor sites. This finding led to the extraction and identification of certain natural compounds that occupy the morphine receptor sites in the brains of mice. When these natural compounds were analyzed, it was apparent, as Dr. Richard Restak, a Washington, D. C., neurologist told me in summing up his recently published interpretation of the process, that "The body manufactures its own opiates."

Scientists in the field now believe that many drugs act on receptor sites, which are located in the cells of the brain and in other organs of the body. The active ingredient of the introduced drug undergoes a chemical reaction within the receptor site. The result of this reaction in some way cures or alleviates the condition being treated.

Further experimentation in this area may yield clues to some of mankind's most intractable problems — pain, drug addiction, and mental illness. It may even be possible for psychiatrists to find a key to schizophrenia in abnormalities or deficiencies in brain receptors.

Medical science, it would seem, has come a long way since Sertürner released morphine from the opium poppy. But nature has always been slow to reveal her secrets, as investigators have learned through centuries of battling the great scourges.

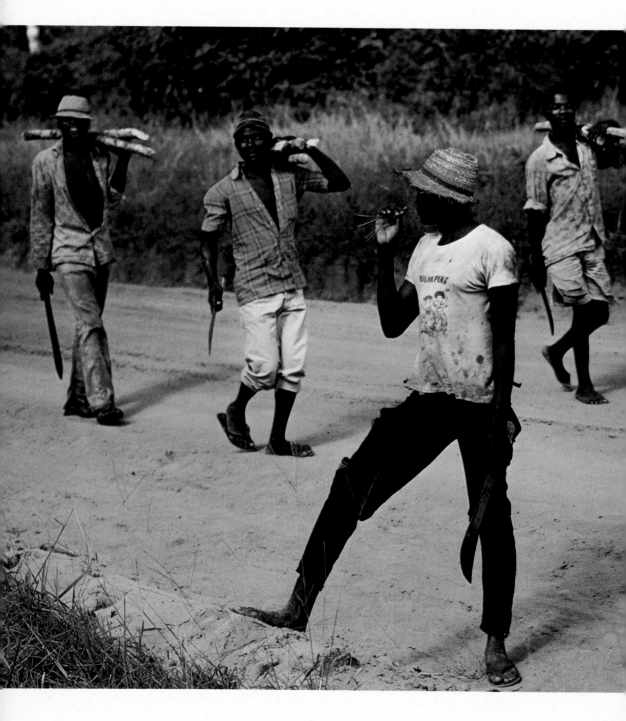

Global search for a cancer cure focuses on Kenya's Shimba Hills, where workers cut vine-like Maytenus buchananii. *Workmen then carry the stems to a waiting vehicle. One of more than 25,000 plant species screened in a U. S. Government program,* Maytenus *may prove useful against cancer.*

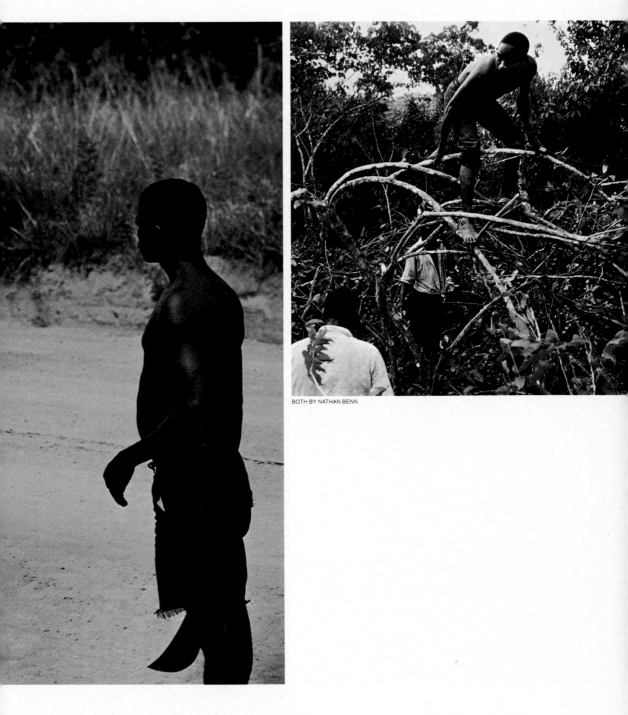

BOTH BY NATHAN BENN

111

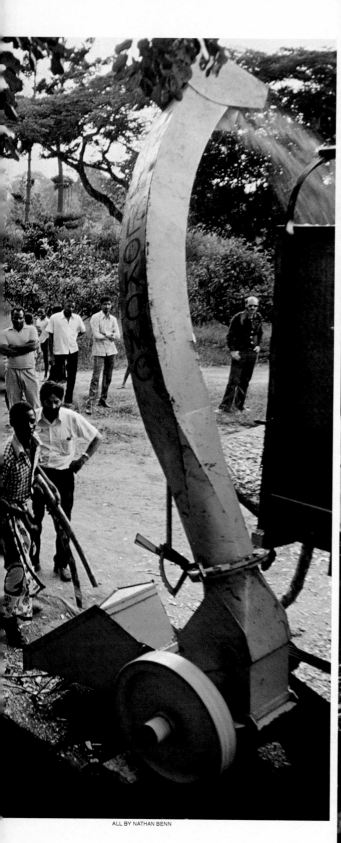

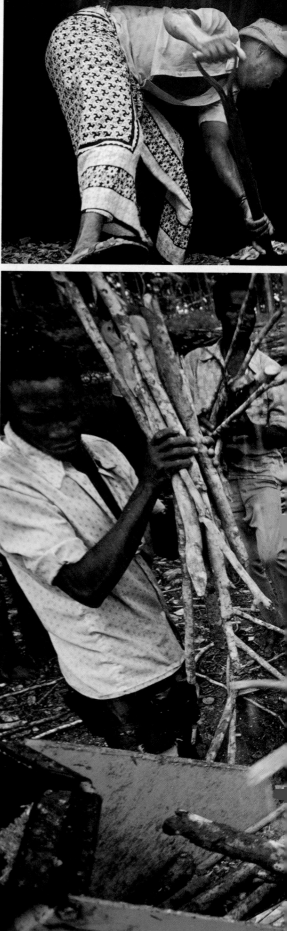

ALL BY NATHAN BENN

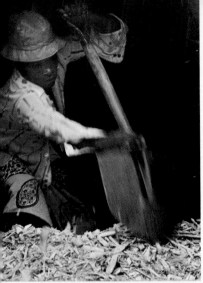

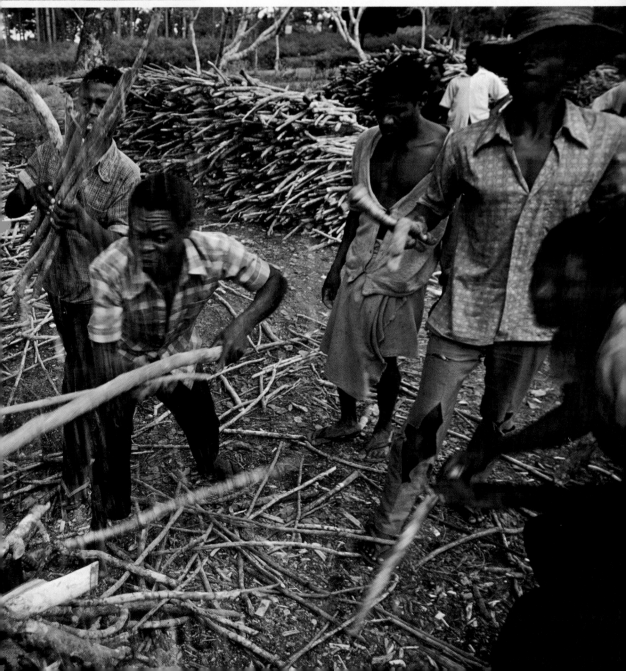

Bits of Maytenus *shower from a wood chipper fed by workers in Kenya. During a cloudburst, two men (left) distribute the chips in a truck. The U. S. Department of Agriculture, working with the National Cancer Institute, harvested some 60,000 pounds of the species for shipment to the U. S. One type of* Maytenus, *says Robert E. Perdue, Jr., botanist in charge of the collection process, forms "part of an African herbal remedy used to treat conditions symptomatic of cancer."*

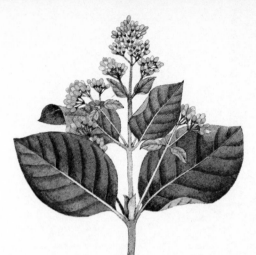

Ancient Scourges Held at Bay

ABOUT THE YEAR 1575, a Spanish physician named Nicolás Monardes wrote a book that was translated under the exuberant title, *Joyfull Newes out of the Newe Founde Worlde*. Its pages contained descriptions and uses of the astonishing variety of medicinal plants then arriving in Europe from the Western Hemisphere. These plants attracted nearly as much attention as the hoards of gold carried in Spanish galleons.

Dr. Monardes wrote that "our Occidentall Indias doeth sende unto us many Trees, Plantes, Herbes, Rootes, Joices, Gummes, Fruites . . . that are of greate medicinall vertues." Among those he listed are many whose "vertues" are still appreciated. One is copal, or sweet gum, an Aztec incense and medication that the Indians applied hot to the cheek for toothache, and which we continue to use for the same purpose today.

The many uses to which Peruvian Indians put "the hearbe . . . they doe call the Coca" fascinated Monardes. They not only chewed its leaves for the pleasant taste, but also mixed them with lime and rolled them into balls to suck for sustenance on long treks through the towering Andes. "These little Bawles dooe take [away] the hunger and thurste," he wrote wonderingly. And he would have been even more amazed

Searching for victims of leprosy, a medical assistant questions a villager in the Central African Republic. In the fight against such dread diseases, health officials battle fear and ignorance, as well as illness.

CINCHONA (ABOVE)

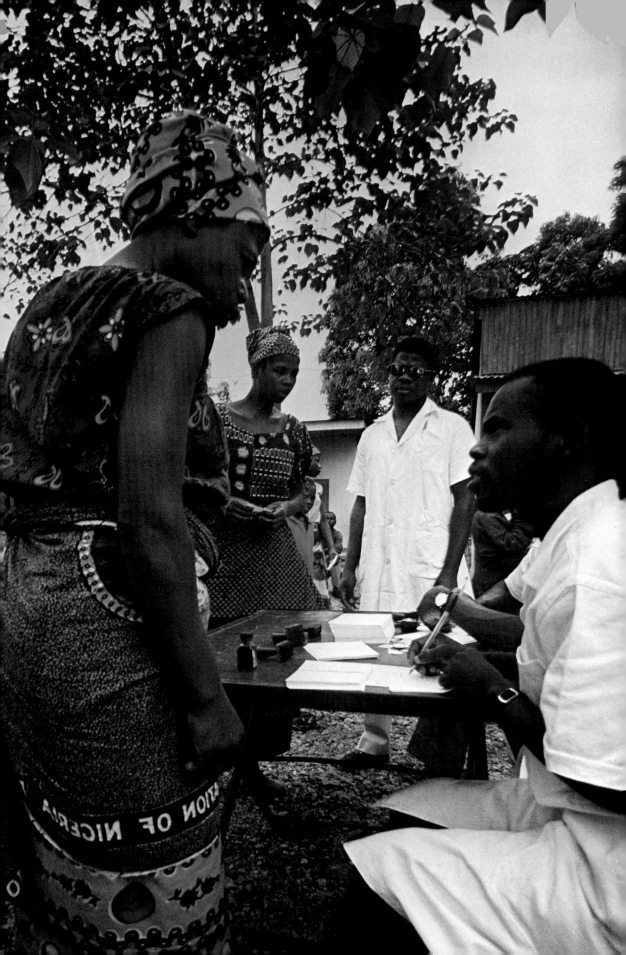

could he have foreseen that some day the same coca would yield a pain-killing substance called cocaine.

More interesting than coca to the drug dealers of Europe was the sassafras tree, which Monardes described as one of "great excellencies." A tea made from its "woodd and roote," he wrote, was used by the Indians of Florida to heal "greevous and variable deseases." They had told French settlers about it, and the French had passed the word on to the Spanish, who were drinking the tea, he said, with "merveilous effectes" against the constant agues, or malaria, suffered from "the naughtie meates and drinkyng of the rawe waters, and slepyng in the dewes." So high was the regard for the "ague tree" that its dried bark became an instant trade success in Europe. By 1618, sassafras was listed in the *Pharmacopoeia Londinensis,* and it was official in the *U. S. Pharmacopoeia* from 1820 to 1926, and in the *National Formulary* until 1965.

But Dr. Monardes missed the real malaria tree—the *Cinchona succirubra,* whose bark would give the world its first effective remedy for the ancient curse that has killed more people than any other disease. Malaria is a debilitating illness, whose alternating cycles of chills and fever lead eventually to a state of shock and, if unchecked, to death.

As a physician, Hippocrates knew malaria's symptoms in the fifth century before Christ. He even correctly identified the different types of attacks that occur daily and those that occur every third or fourth day. Great armies, from ancient times on, have been decimated by this enemy. Kings and queens paid royal fees in attempts to rid themselves of the disease's excruciating aches and pains. Rome and its surrounding marshy areas were feared for centuries as one of the regions of the world most vulnerable to malaria. In the United States, the young capital at Washington suffered annual visitations of malaria, as did many sections of the new nation.

When early Spanish explorers reached the eastern slopes of the Andes, they saw growing there a magnificent flowering evergreen — the cinchona. Its use was first recorded in a religious book written in 1633 by an Augustinian monk named Calancha of Peru. The author wrote of "the fever tree [that] produced miraculous results." It cured fevers, he explained, with a powder made from the bark "amounting to the weight of two small silver coins and given as a beverage."

The bark of this Peruvian tree was destined to make medical history. It was called Jesuits' bark, after missionary priests of that order began shipping it to Europe about 1640. Though die-hard physicians, pharmacists, and religious opponents denounced its distribution as a Papist plot to murder Protestants, thousands of malaria victims swallowed the bitter tea. They gained relief, and sometimes cure.

As overseas trade in raw cinchona burgeoned, two French chemists discovered the secret of its effectivenesss in an active alkaloid they isolated from the bark in September 1820. They called it "quinine," for an old

Inca term, *quina-quina,* or bark of barks, and generously gave it to the world without claiming patent rights.

As early as 1823, the first quinine factory in the United States opened in Philadelphia to meet the demand. In the 1830's, Dr. John Sappington of Arrow Rock, Missouri, began mixing his own "anti-fever" pills, with which distributors supplied much of the Mississippi River Valley. Rival practitioners grumbled, but historians now praise the good doctor for eliminating malaria in a large section of the Midwest.

The worldwide success of quinine brought with it the horrifying specter of vanishing bark supplies. During the first two centuries following its discovery, cinchona bark had been taken almost entirely from the Loja region near Peru's northern border with Ecuador—by the simple process of felling the trees without replanting. So wasteful was this method that by 1850 the consuming nations were forced to seek alternate sources.

After decades of exploration and bitter international rivalry for world markets, the English botanist Richard Spruce discovered the red-bark cinchona in the Andes of Ecuador in 1860. Out of the sturdy root stock of this *succirubra* and its hybrids came a tree combining reliability with the highest quinine yield known.

The way was now clear for large-scale cultivation of these trees, but still no one knew what caused the disease. It was not until 1880 that a French army surgeon in North Africa, Alphonse Laveran, described a parasitic organism he saw through his microscope as the malaria agent. Other investigators followed the trail of the parasite carrier, or vector. In 1898, Sir Ronald Ross, a British bacteriologist in the Indian health service, spotlighted the culprit as the female anopheles mosquito.

Since then, the battle has been fought on many fronts and with many weapons, as the mosquitoes developed defenses against each new assault. At the Center for Disease Control in Atlanta, Georgia, I checked with Dr. Geoffrey M. Jeffery of the Bureau of Tropical Diseases, U. S. Public Health Service. Dr. Jeffery has been involved with malaria research for more than 30 years, entering the Public Health Service during World War II to work on the malaria-control program at U. S. military camps. Later, he continued to study malaria and associated diseases in the Tennessee River Valley and elsewhere in the United States, Puerto Rico, and, most recently, El Salvador.

When we met, I found a tall, pleasant man with an ascetic face, who hopes that the goal of malaria eradication may be reached eventually, "whether in fifteen or a hundred years," he said. "There have been many disappointments in the past, and there will doubtless be more.

"After Ross's discovery of the anopheles *(Continued on page 124)*

Overleaf: English botanist Richard Spruce collects seeds from cinchona trees during an 1860 expedition to Ecuador. Quinine extracted from cinchona bark still alleviates malaria—mankind's most deadly disease.

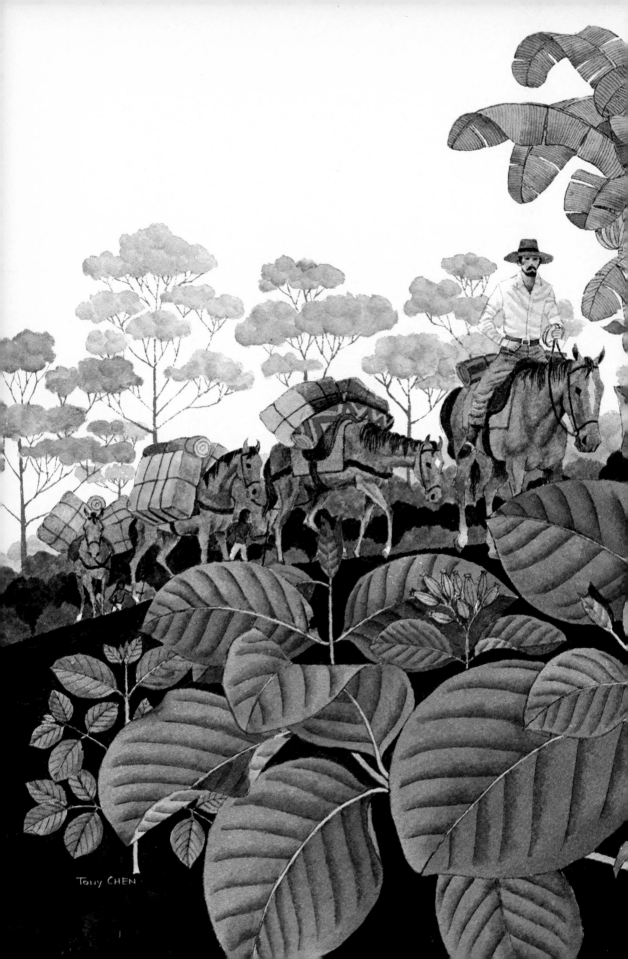

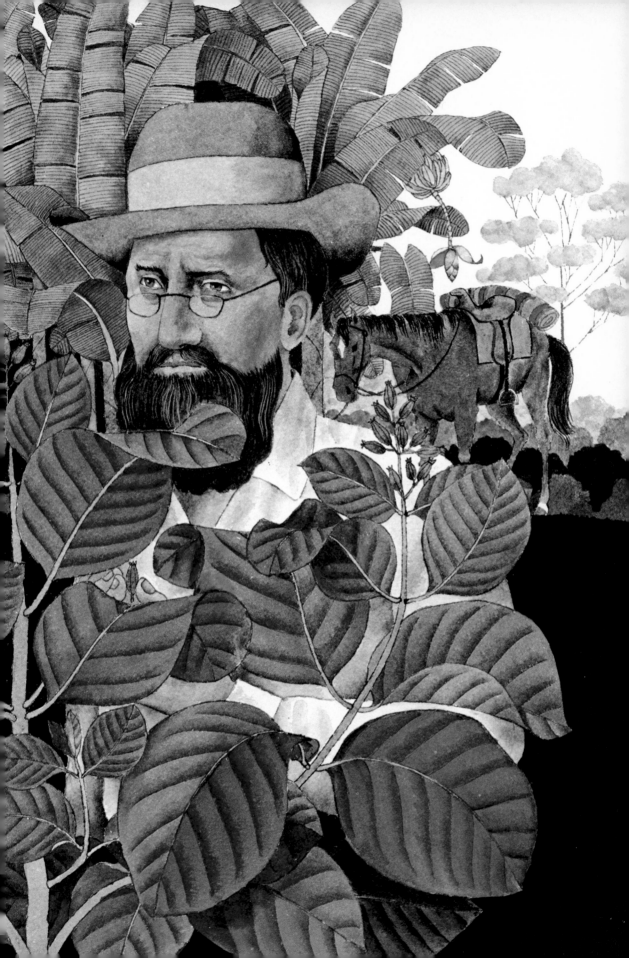

Protected by antimalarial drugs, a researcher in El Salvador sits shirtless at dusk to attract mosquitoes. As they alight, his colleague collects them to determine the effectiveness of an experiment in mosquito control. Female mosquitoes of the genus Anopheles—such as the one below engorged with blood—transmit malaria; controlling these insects means controlling the disease. Malaria, with its cycles of high fever and severe chills, weakens victims and can eventually kill them. In this experiment, scientists of the U. S. Department of Agriculture and the Public Health Service—working with the government of El Salvador—alter the natural reproductive cycle of the mosquito. They breed the insects, separate the males and sterilize them, and then release them. If a female mates with a sterile male the eggs remain infertile and do not hatch. Earlier tests indicated a substantial reduction in the local mosquito population.

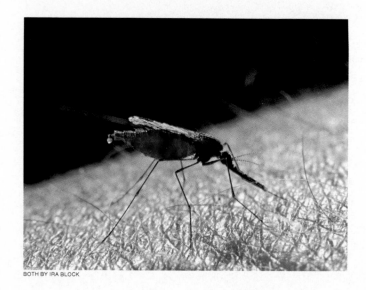

BOTH BY IRA BLOCK

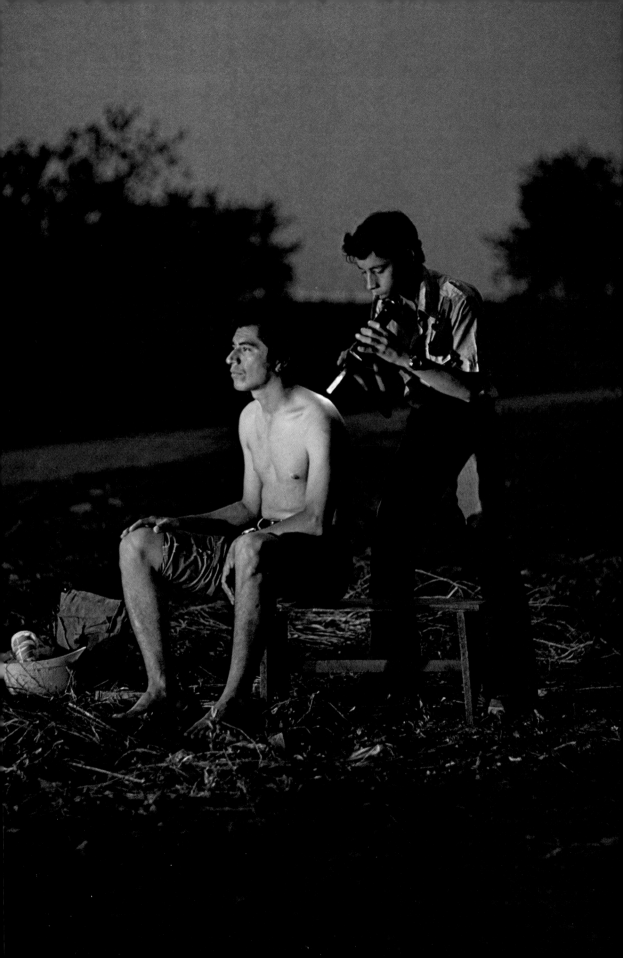

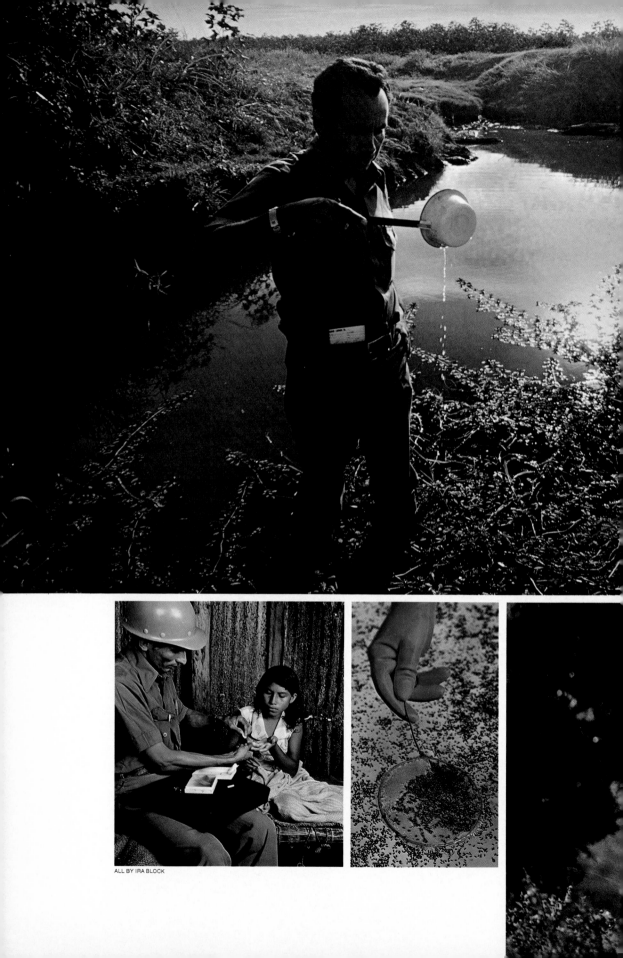

ALL BY IRA BLOCK

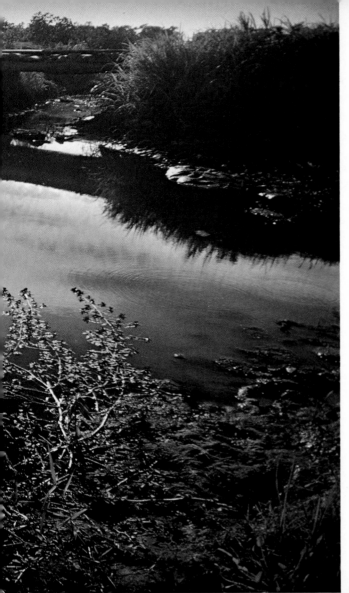

Snapping open a carrying box (below), an employee of the Department of Agriculture releases a thousand sterile male mosquitoes in El Salvador. A chemical bath like the one at center below sterilized the insects during their pupal stage. Careful observations enabled the researchers to evaluate the success of their battle against malaria. Holding a dipper, a field supervisor (left) examines pond water for mosquito larvae and pupae. Another worker (lower, left) takes a blood smear from a woman's fingertip to check her for malaria.

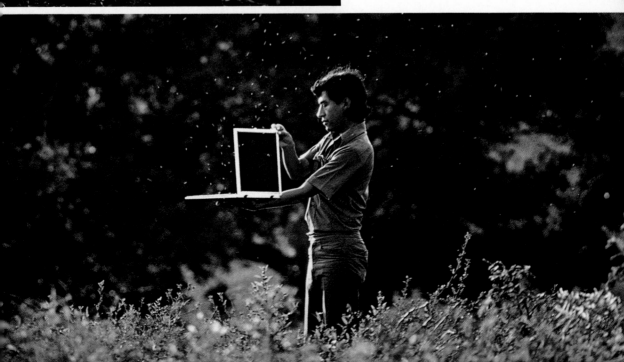

carrier, and on through the First World War," he said, "there was great optimism that the problem could be solved by two steps: first, draining mosquito breeding areas and killing the larvae in the water, and then putting screens on houses and spraying inside with insecticides. Also, we had quinine as a specific treatment—a rare advantage against any disease.

"But malaria was not that easily conquered," he went on. "There are many species of the genus *Anopheles,* with differing habits to cope with. Quinine itself presents difficulties; it has a bitter taste and often causes dizziness and a ringing sensation in the ears. So synthetic drugs were developed as early as the 1920's to supplement and supplant it. One of the big problems we face now is that the parasites in some parts of the world have become resistant to the synthetic drugs. As a result, quinine again is an effective alternative drug, either alone or in combination with synthetics. This practice has been followed successfully in treating the dangerous Viet Nam type of falciparum malaria."

Still, malaria the killer is far from being banished from the earth. True, it has been eradicated in the United States as an endemic disease, though theoretically it could be reintroduced. But in Central and South America, Africa, and the Far and Middle East, it has actually increased. Every year an estimated million and a half people die of it.

Malaria fighters continue to try new techniques. One, used in El Salvador, involves releasing sterile anopheles males into areas affected by malaria. Since the disease-carrying females mate only once, the object is to reduce offspring by increasing the number of sterile males present. Another promising technique is to stock the waters where mosquitoes breed with insect-eating fish and other predators.

"But the overall need," said Dr. Jeffery, "is for more laboratory research and field training on a variety of measures—including the development of a malaria-preventing vaccine. Together, these steps may take us closer to realizing the dream of eradicating mankind's primary infectious disease. To have had even a small part in such a victory would be reward enough for a lifetime of effort."

Unlike malaria, smallpox—another worldwide pestilence feared and loathed throughout history—is today making its last stand. Such is the belief, at least, of those people in the World Health Organization engaged in the remarkably successful eradication program, which is now nearing completion after ten years of prodigious effort.

At the Bureau of Smallpox Eradication—also a part of the Atlanta Center for Disease Control—I learned from Dr. Stanley Foster how the international campaign against smallpox was organized and waged. He had spent eight of the program's ten years as a medical officer in some of the worst trouble spots of Africa and Asia.

"To start at the present and work back," said Dr. Foster, "we had hoped that the few cases of smallpox reported in Ethiopia in the summer of 1976 would be the last ones, and that the outbreak could be quickly and locally contained. Unfortunately, the disease escaped to Mogadishu, the capital of Somalia, and later to northeast Kenya. The transmission now seems to have been interrupted in Ethiopia, but as long as there is one case, it remains a threat to the entire world."

And that threat is frighteningly awesome. Smallpox is a highly contagious disease characterized by high fever and the eruption of itching and burning pustules. It leaves the skin pitted and scarred—and can kill.

To appreciate the magnitude of the task achieved in reducing the old scourge of smallpox to its present minuscule state, consider the many centuries that it decimated populations everywhere. Evidence of the ravages of this disease has been found in the earliest records of China and India, and the pockmarked mummy of Ramesses V suggests that the death of this Egyptian pharaoh in 1160 B.C. was possibly due to it. Ancient Greece and Rome seem to have been spared the devastating pestilence, but it was known in Europe in the 6th century A.D. In 910, the Persian physician Rhazes published the first precise description of it in *A Treatise On the Small Pox and Measles*.

By the 16th and 17th centuries, smallpox epidemics were racing across Europe and Asia and becoming even more terrifying, because of the disfigurement and high death toll, than that other mass destroyer, the bubonic plague. After the discovery of the New World, colonists brought the white man's diseases, and smallpox struck with special ferocity at the Indians, who had no immunity to it.

Governor William Bradford of Massachusetts wrote in the *History of Plimoth Plantation* of an epidemic that spread in 1634. "This spring, also, those Indeans that lived aboute their trading house there fell sick of the small poxe, and dyed most miserably . . . they fall into a lamentable condition. . . . not able to help [one] another; no, not to make a fire, nor to fetch a litle water to drink nor any to burie the dead."

Yet a remedy was known even then, not to cure the disease—there is still no cure once it has been contracted—but to develop immunity and prevent its spread. In a sense, it was nature's own method, fighting illness with illness.

Rural people, living with nature, had used this folk remedy in Asia and Europe for many centuries. The technique, crude but effective, was simply to take the scabs or the material from the pimple-like pustules of a smallpox victim and make contact with an open scratch in the skin of the healthy person. If successful, only a mild case developed, giving lifetime immunity. Even when a severe case or an occasional death resulted, supporters of the method preferred it to taking a chance on the many fatalities that accompanied the unchecked disease.

This primitive form of inoculation was called variolation, and received its first serious trial in the American Colonies during Boston's deadly smallpox epidemic of 1721. But so intense was the fear of it that only one physician, Dr. Zabdiel Boylston, braved the opposition of other doctors and the mob violence of frantic citizens to practice it. Dr. Boylston inoculated his own son, who survived. Later, Boylston informed the Royal Society of London that deaths from his induced cases numbered, proportionately, only a small fraction of those caused by natural infection.

Despite its relative success in Boston, variolation was still furiously debated during the American Revolution, when smallpox was one of the major problems of the army and of the civilian populations. George Washington was fortunately immune, having had a mild case of the disease on a trip to the Caribbean as a youth. He also saw to it that Martha was inoculated; Mrs. Washington seemed to react "favourably . . . very few pustules," he remarked in a letter to his brother, John Augustine.

The great variolation controversy finally died a natural death in most parts of the world after Edward Jenner, an English physician with a country practice in Gloucestershire, introduced his cowpox vaccination in 1798. Dr. Jenner had first thought of the procedure in the 1770's when he noticed that milkmaids infected by a mild animal disease called cowpox seemed immune to smallpox. Following his hunch, he studied and experimented, and, in 1789, vaccinated his healthy young son with matter from the milder pox. The infection produced a light case, and made him immune in subsequent exposure to smallpox.

A few years later, when cowpox again broke out in his region, Dr. Jenner demonstrated his theory once more by vaccinating an eight-year-old boy with matter from cowpox pustules. This boy also was protected from smallpox. Although Jenner's thesis initially met with some distrust and skepticism, it was accepted generally by most of the medical profession in Europe and America.

"Jenner gave us the key to global eradication of smallpox," said Dr. Foster, as we talked of the problems and achievements of the campaign by the World Health Organization. "At present this disease is probably the only major one that can be completely eradicated. It can be diagnosed without laboratory tests; its infectious period is short—maybe two to three weeks; only persons in the rash stage of the disease can spread it; vaccination is simple and inexpensive; and immunity—once obtained—is long-lasting. But, of course, there were many obstacles to overcome.

"At the end of World War II, smallpox was endemic in almost every country. Then, during the postwar recovery period, successful vaccination programs eliminated the disease or brought it under control in most countries except in tropical areas of Asia, Africa, and South America. In the United States, for instance, the last reported case occurred in 1949.

"There were technological improvements, too, in the old vaccines and methods of injection," Dr. Foster continued. "The virus, grown under sterile conditions in the skin of live calves or in the membrane of chicken embryos, was removed at the time of maximum potency and made into heat-stable, freeze-dried vaccine. The use of jet injectors and forked needles speeded up the process and improved the rate of effectiveness from 50 to 98 percent. So the stage was set for WHO to inaugurate its ambitious ten-year program to wipe smallpox from the face of the globe."

From Dr. Foster I learned that the project was proposed largely at the instigation of the Soviet Union and the United States. These two countries were joined by others to provide manpower, money, and vaccine to assist the infected nations in ridding themselves of smallpox. This cooperation was invaluable to the success of the program, he said. During the two years that he was in charge of activities in Bangladesh, representatives of 28 different nations worked together. No less extraordinary was the personal dedication of both the leaders and the village-level health teams who labored under hard and hazardous conditions ranging from miserable weather to inadequate food to warfare.

But the most important factor in the ultimate success of the program, Dr. Foster said, was changing the original system of mass vaccination to one called "surveillance and containment." Mass vaccination had often missed uncooperative groups and permitted the disease to escape. The strategy adopted was to search in homes and markets and to offer rewards for finding active cases. The sick people were then isolated and all who had been in contact with them were vaccinated. This practice was especially effective in India and Bangladesh, where density of population and movement between village and city made for rapid spread of the disease.

"Out of it all," he concluded, "came even more than the virtual eradication of a major cause of human suffering. We learned how to use local people effectively in field campaigns against other ravaging diseases such as malaria and measles. We saw the power of cooperation between East and West, between developed and developing nations. With it may come the realization that we live in one global village, in which health is everybody's problem."

The sun was just breaking through the clouds when I arrived at the U. S. Public Health Service Hospital at Carville, Louisiana, after a short plane ride from Atlanta to the Baton Rouge airport, and a 25-mile drive through a heavy rainstorm. Later, after I had had a chance to tour the hospital and recreational facilities available to leprosy patients and to talk with doctors who treat them, the sunshine following the storm seemed to me to symbolize the light into which this disease has finally begun to emerge from misunderstanding and prejudice.

Caused by bacteria, leprosy may produce spots on the skin and damage nerve cells. Loss of feeling follows, and eventually the extremities suffer injuries and infections, which can lead (Continued on page 134)

Overleaf: Edward Jenner scrapes matter from pustules on a Gloucestershire milkmaid mildly ill with cowpox. A vaccine of the material, the English physician found in the late 18th century, protected against smallpox.

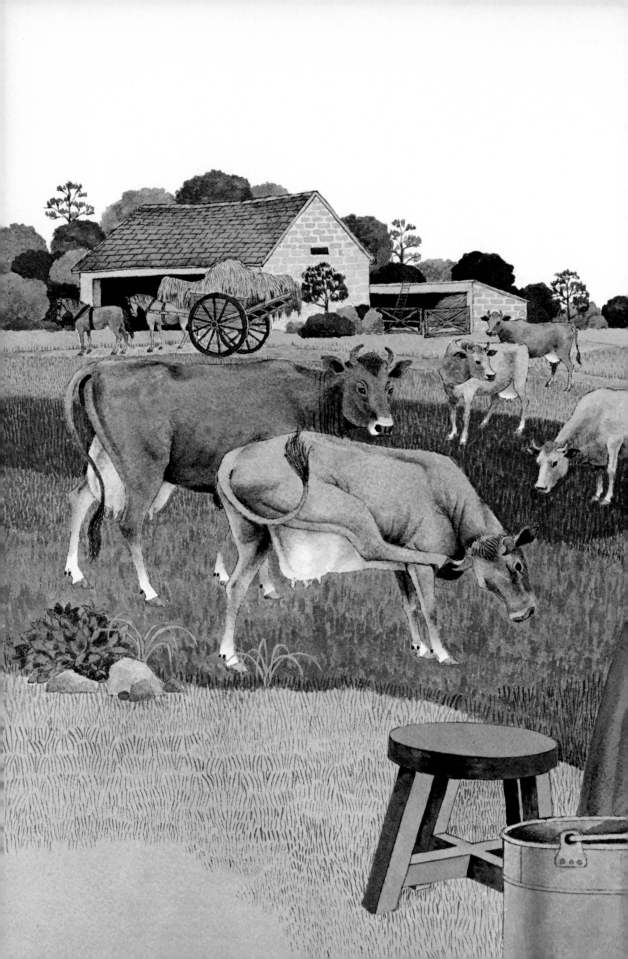

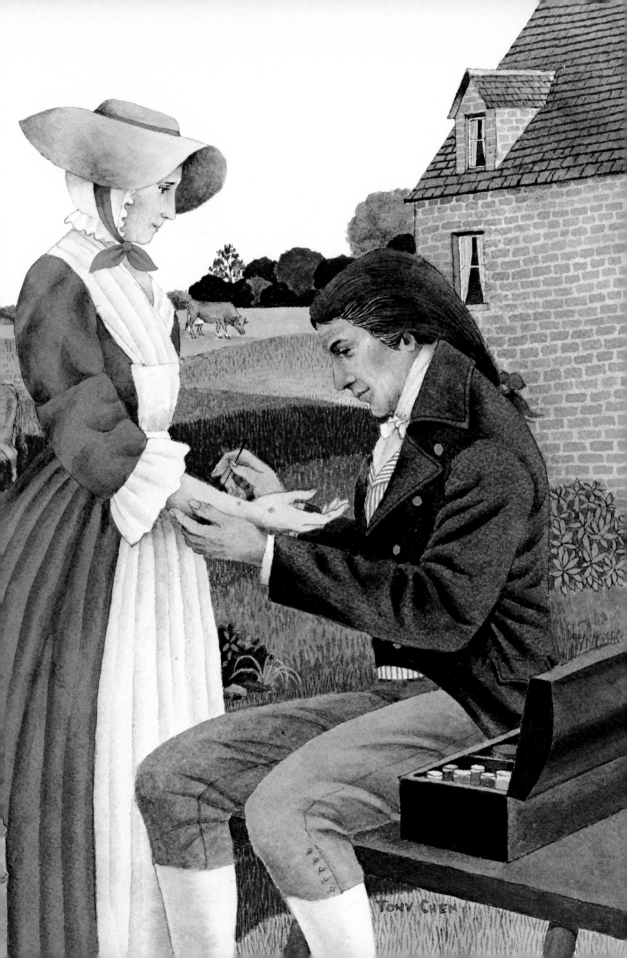

Helicopter of a smallpox surveillance team touches down near a district medical office after visiting a remote village in the mountains of Ethiopia — possibly one of the last regions in the world where the disease exists. A medical worker (below) checks the vaccination scar on a child. Alert for any new cases of the disease, he shows villagers a picture of a smallpox victim, then asks if they have seen anyone with a similar illness.

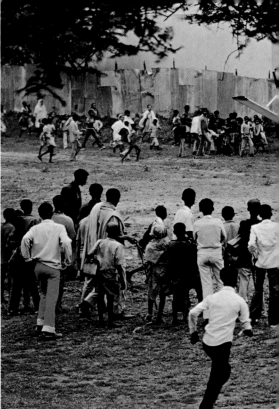

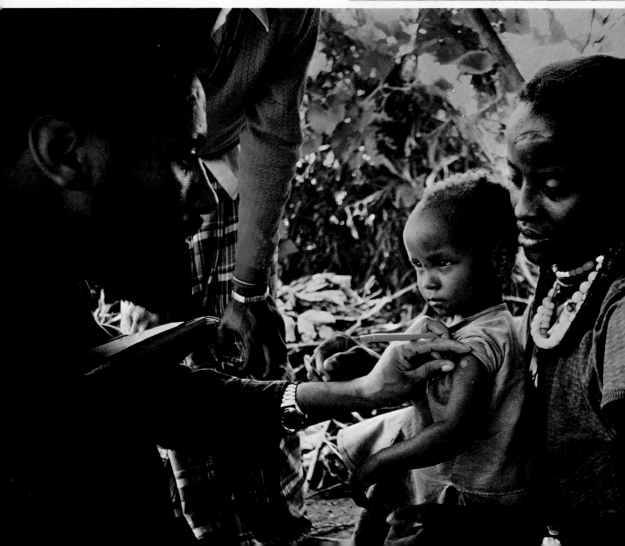

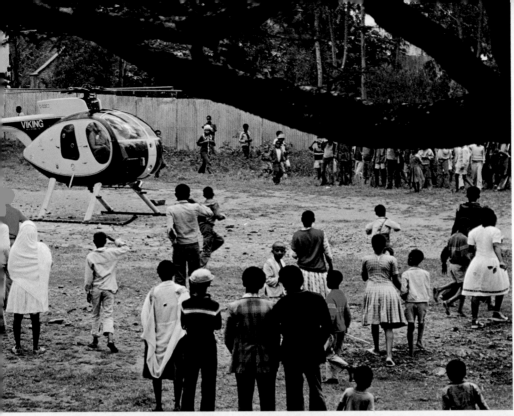

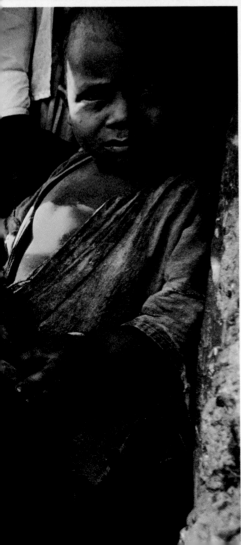

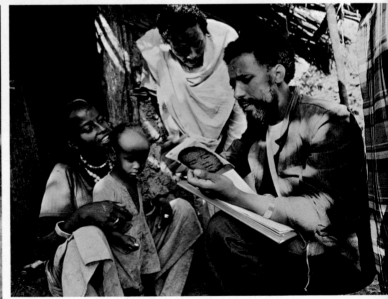

ALL BY MARION KAPLAN

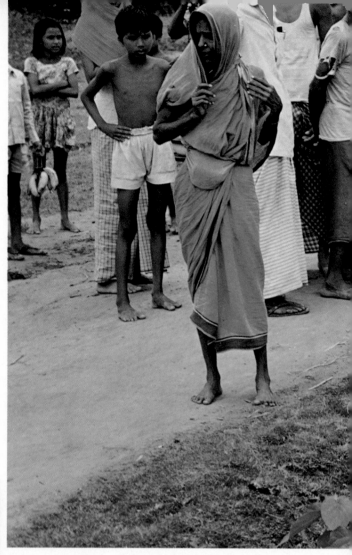

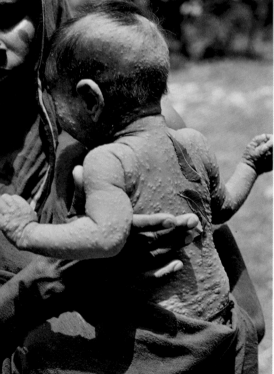

Assisting a man stricken with smallpox, an English physician working for the World Health Organization helps him to an isolation hut in

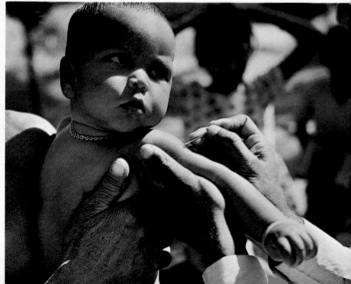

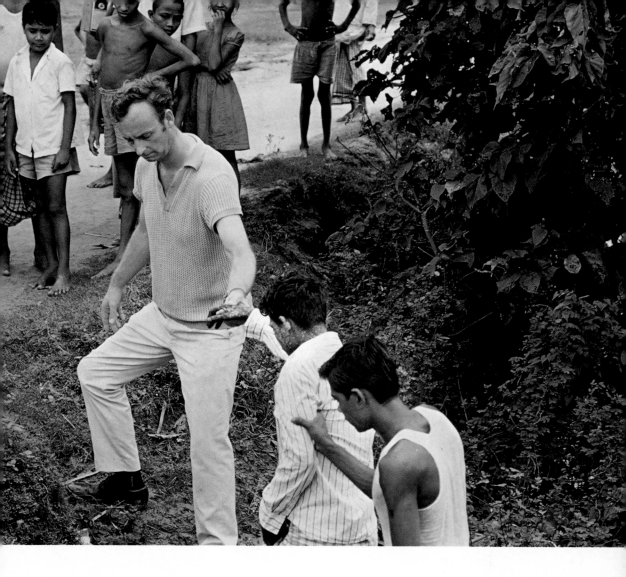

Bangladesh. Other workers will immunize anyone the patient may have infected. The forked needle and the jet gun (below) serve as the major means of vaccinating worldwide. Opposite: Neem leaves, Bangladesh villagers believe, relieve the discomfort of smallpox.

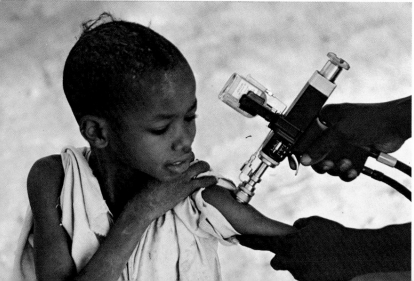

to loss of hands and feet. The disease has been around for a long time. Dr. Stanley G. Browne, who heads the Leprosy Study Center in London, has traced its existence in India to 600 B.C. Although the Bible often refers to "leprosy," this is "a ritualistic term denoting defilement or uncleanness," writes Dr. Browne in his book, *Leprosy in the Bible*. It meant "a pathological condition . . . mentioned in a context of illness and affliction. . . ."

Whatever the true ailment of an unfortunate person thought to have leprosy, he was cruelly treated in the past, especially in medieval days. "In countries of southern Europe, and to a much lesser extent in England, the infamous 'lepers mass' was celebrated," says Dr. Browne. Hooded and shrouded, these victims were forbidden "to enter church, marketplaces, the mill, the bakehouse, the assembly of the people. . ." without their "leper uniform." Those wishing to observe mass were forced to remain outside and peer through what were called "squint windows."

As old as leprosy are the folklore medicines that have been used to fight it. Most of these treatments are obviously fanciful, such as those listed in John Wesley's book, *Primitive Remedies,* which was standard as late as the 18th century. In it he suggested mixtures that included powdered brimstone, houseleeks, and celery whey—and advised sufferers to "wash in the sea often and long."

One ancient plant product, however, turned out to have real value in treating leprosy. It was an acrid oil from the seeds of the rare chaulmoogra tree, which grows in Asia. From time beyond memory, patrons of Eastern bazaars have been buying such seeds to heal skin lesions, especially those of leprosy. A legend dating to pre-Buddhist times tells of a Burmese king who contracted leprosy and exiled himself to the jungle. He lived there in a hollow tree and ate the fruits and leaves of the chaulmoogra. Eventually the diet cured him, and he returned to his throne.

In the real world, botanical knowledge supported legend and custom when the great 16th-century Chinese naturalist, Li Shih-chen, confirmed the value of chaulmoogra oil in treating leprosy. But broad interest in its use was delayed for several more centuries, partly because of the problem of identifying the correct species of tree, and partly because of the nausea that follows ingestion of the raw oil.

British scientists refined the oil in 1904. Sixteen years later, Dr. David Fairchild, then head of the U. S. Department of Agriculture's Office of Foreign Seed and Plant Introduction, arranged a government expedition to Southeast Asia to locate a large stand of the elusive trees. For the job, he engaged an Austrian-born, Chinese-speaking botanist named Joseph Rock of the University of Hawaii.

Dr. Rock told the story of his mission in the March 1922 NATIONAL GEOGRAPHIC. During his trip, he encountered bandits and man-eating tigers before finally reaching his goal in a thick growth of the chaulmoogra species *Taraktogenos Kurzii* in northeast Burma. He extracted the precious seeds from the big, orange-like fruit of the tree and shipped them to Hawaii for cultivation. In time, the mature trees began yielding a high-grade oil that would introduce the only medically accepted leprosy treatment available for the next 20 years.

On my visit to the Carville hospital, I met Sister Laura Stricker, who has worked there for half a century, and who administered some of the first doses of chaulmoogra oil. "In the early days, chaulmoogra oil was all we had," she said. "It was shipped to us by a distributor who ordered it from India. It was in its raw state then, and many patients couldn't tolerate the nausea it caused, or the pain of injection. Also, it was slow-acting. Sometimes years would pass before there was noticeable improvement."

I learned more about the disease itself when I talked with Dr. Robert R. Jacobson, Chief of Medicine at the hospital. "Leprosy—which is properly called Hansen's disease—primarily attacks the skin and peripheral nerves. It is not very communicable, especially in countries like the United States in which it is not endemic. We have about 325 patients at this hospital, and only those with long-term illnesses choose to stay permanently. Others come and go. The disease is not considered infectious when under treatment, and many people lead normal working lives."

The hospital abandoned the use of chaulmoogra oil in 1947, Dr. Jacobson told me, after five or six years of testing had shown that the newly developed sulfone drugs were more effective. Lately, however, the leprosy bacilli infecting some patients have developed resistance to the sulfone compounds. So the search is on to find other drugs. Some researchers are restudying chaulmoogra oil's hydnocarpic and chaulmoogric acids—both of which have shown activity against leprosy ever since the earliest tests in the 1920's. "Perhaps we may yet find something new and useful in the old chaulmoogra treatment," said Dr. Jacobson.

Meanwhile, the hospital is carrying on another phase of its official mission—the surgical repair of patients severely damaged by the disease's progressive destruction of the skin and nerves of the face, hands, and feet. "Until comparatively recently, people deformed by leprosy faced a miserable future," said Dr. Carl D. Enna, chief of the hospital's Surgical Department and Clinical Branch. "Now there is hope, with drugs to control the disease, and surgery to correct or alleviate disfigurements."

Before leaving Carville, I spoke with the hospital director, Dr. John Trautman, about the present and future of leprosy as a world problem. "Estimates of its incidence range anywhere from 12 to 20 million," he said, "with a very high percentage reported from India and central Africa. In the United States, the disease is more or less under control, but in undeveloped countries, figures are rising at a disturbing rate. We can only keep on working, and keep on hoping."

After all, other diseases have given way to unexpected breakthroughs. Heart failure, for one, lost some of its terror when an 18th-century doctor discovered a plant to treat dropsy.

135

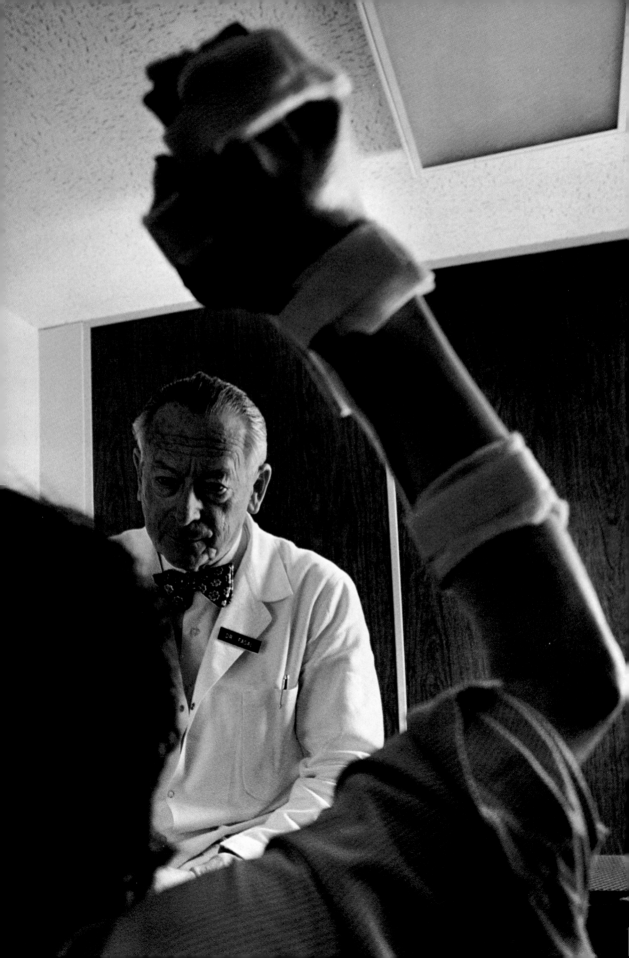

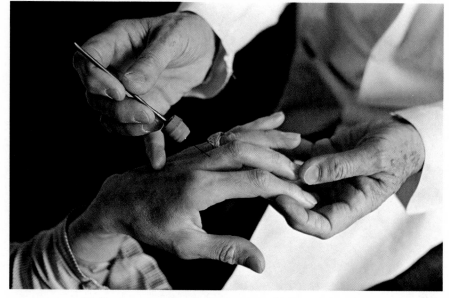

His arm raised by a splint to assist healing, a patient with leprosy, or Hansen's disease, talks with Dr. Paul Fasal at the Public Health Service Hospital in San Francisco. A surgeon there operated to restore the use of the hand. Today, many leprosy victims can lead normal lives with regular outpatient treatment. Leprosy can attack many organs—including nerves and skin—and cause impaired feeling. Above, Dr. Fasal tests a patient for sensitivity to touch. Seen through a microscope (below, right), leprosy bacteria dyed red for diagnosis invade the nerve at the right; only a few appear around the blood vessel next to it. A thermogram of a hand shows temperatures as colors—yellow means warmth, blue indicates coolness. The thermogram reveals marked damage to nerves of the little finger; if untreated, the patient may lose it through injury and infection.

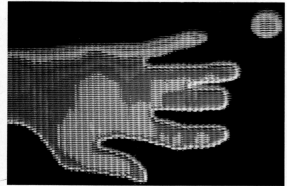
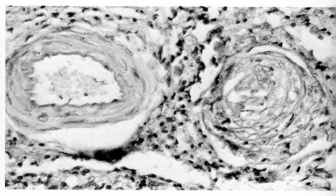

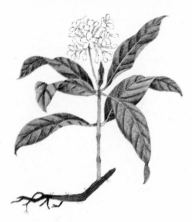

Toward Conquests
of Old Killers

HEARTS AND FLOWERS. Together, they make a combination that is perhaps better suited to a romantic novel than to one of the most momentous advances in medical history. In this landmark case the hearts were ailing, and the flowers were pretty garden blooms called foxgloves. Their connection gave the world its most widely prescribed drugs to stimulate and regulate the human heart.

The man responsible for the medical bonanza was William Withering, a physician who practiced 200 years ago in the pleasant country district of Staffordshire, England. Dr. Withering was a serious-minded young man whose interests ranged from music to mineralogy to botany. Though he had expressed a dislike of botany as a medical student, part of his later courtship of Helene Cookes was to go out into the field and collect wild flowers as subjects for her paintings.

However his botanical knowledge was acquired, Withering was well prepared to take advantage of the circumstances that led to his discovery of the foxglove plant as the source of digitalis. The story began in 1775 when the doctor was practicing in Birmingham. He traveled 60 miles back and forth to the Stafford Infirmary, where he treated indigent patients

Peruvian Indian's cheek bulges with a wad of coca leaves. A mild stimulant and rich source of vitamins and minerals, coca yields the anesthetic cocaine; tests show it may have potential as a treatment for high-altitude sickness.

RAUWOLFIA (ABOVE)

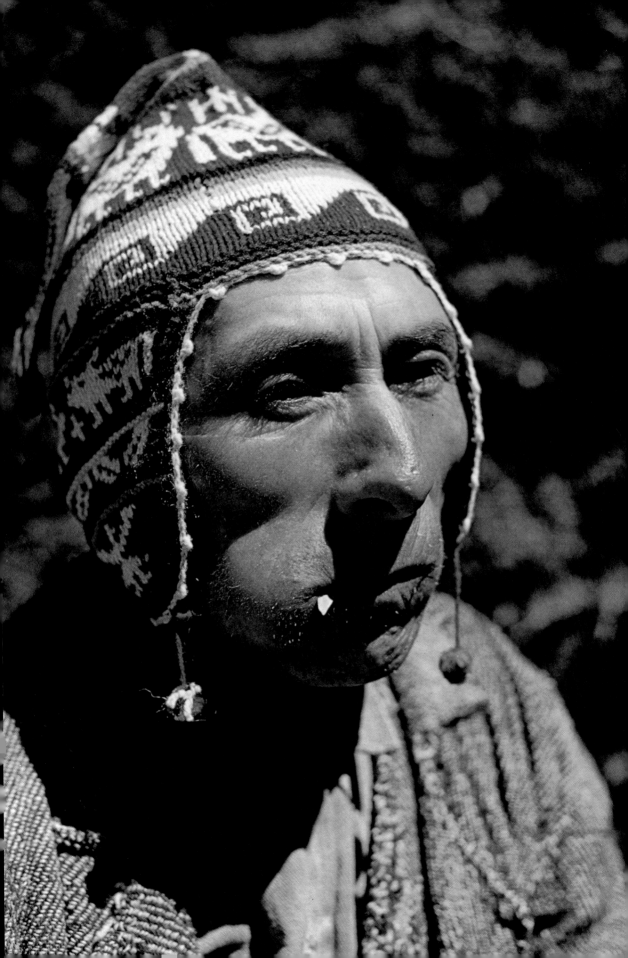

free. During one trip, he agreed to visit a woman along the way who was suffering from dropsy — accumulated water in the chest and abdomen and swelling of the arms, legs, and ankles. He saw her, but felt he could do nothing to save her life. Later, he inquired about her condition and was amazed to find that she had recovered, thanks to a secret herbal recipe provided by an old "wise woman" of Shropshire.

Curious, Dr. Withering obtained from the old lady a sampling of her medicinal plants and proceeded to analyze them. "This medicine was composed of twenty or more different herbs," he wrote of his findings, "but it was not very difficult for one conversant with these subjects to perceive that the active herb could be no other than the Foxglove."

Withering devoted ten years to studying the plant and recording the reactions of each of 163 patients to whom he gave the drug — "successful or otherwise," as he put it honestly in his classic treatise, *An Account of the Foxglove and Some of its Medical Uses.*

He learned that the active ingredient was in the long, green leaves, and discovered that the best time to gather them was when the blossoms were expanding "at the phase of maximal activity." At first he made a decoction of whole leaves; then he turned to a cold-water infusion after concluding that boiling altered their quality. Finally he decided that the most efficient way to process the leaves was to dry them in the sun or in front of a fire and then grind them into dust. "If well dried," he wrote, the leaves "readily rub down to a beautiful green powder."

Most important, Dr. Withering cautiously worked out a safe dosage in dealing with this substance he knew to be highly dangerous, and sometimes lethal, if improperly prepared or administered. "I give to adults from one to three grains of this powder twice a day," he wrote.

Like all physicians of his time, Withering believed that dropsy was a disease in itself, rather than the symptom of a failing heart, as it later came to be recognized. But his contribution to medical progress was no less significant because of that. Digitalis and other preparations born of his genius continue to lead in treating heart failure by strengthening and improving the tone of the heart muscle, regulating the blood flow, and bringing about a slower but stronger heartbeat.

To some extent, powdered leaves of digitalis are still given in pill, capsule, or tablet form. In fact, some physicians prefer the natural product because of its slower effect. On the other hand, if rapid relief is essential, heart specialists can now call on crystalline glycosides extracted from two different forms of digitalis. One is digitoxin, which was first found in 1869, but not followed up chemically and pharmaceutically until the 1920's. The other is digoxin, isolated in 1930.

Both drugs can save lives, but doctors treat digitoxin with wary respect and administer it in minute quantities since it is a perilously poisonous substance. Digoxin, because of its quicker elimination in case of toxic effects, has much wider use.

Just how far stretches the bright beam of Dr. Withering's painstaking work with the common garden foxglove can be measured today by a single statistic from a comprehensive new book, *Medical Botany, Plants Affecting Man's Health,* by Walter H. Lewis and Memory P. F. Elvin-Lewis. In the United States alone, they report, "more than 3 million cardiac sufferers . . . routinely use the glycoside digoxin. . . ."

For such an important medicinal plant, however, foxglove has a surprisingly vague prehistory. It was mentioned as early as 1250 in records of Welsh physicians, but without details. In *The Herball,* John Gerard suggested that when "boiled in water or wine, and drunken, [it] doth cut and consume the thicke toughnesse of A grosse and slimie flegme and naughtie humours. . . ." Even so, he qualified his remarks by saying that foxgloves are "bitter . . . hot and drie, with a certain kinde of clensing qualitie . . . yet are they of no use . . . amongst medicines." Accounts from country folk, such as the woman Withering interviewed, were the first clues to the plant's value.

Nature, however, has long offered many other cardiac aids from her medicine cabinet, some of which still meet specific needs. Squill, a large bulbous root found in lands along the Mediterranean, is one of the most ancient. It was listed in the Ebers Papyrus, and Hippocrates used it against ulcers and empyema—fluid in a body cavity.

Dioscorides put it in prescriptions to "mollify the belly," and also described a method of preparing a "vinegar of Squills" with oil and wine as a heart tonic that is still official in the *British Pharmacopoeia.*

Squill entered the world of modern medicine in 1879 with the scientific demonstration by E. von Jarmersted of Germany that it contained an active heart glycoside, later separated into three bitter glycosidic substances. The therapeutic action of squill is generally considered to be similar to that of digitalis, but with the disadvantage of being more irritating to the gastrointestinal tract.

Along with several other natural drugs that act strongly on the heart, squill has a more sinister side among African and South American tribes as a poison for arrows. The Nvika people in Tanzania smear arrows with a paste of dried and pounded squill so poisonous that animals or humans are said to die within three hours after being struck.

Equally virulent is ouabain, an active heart glycoside found in the seeds of a tropical African vine. Despite its toxicity, ouabain is medically prized as a lifesaver in emergency therapy. Given intravenously, it acts on the heart within five minutes and is effective   *(Continued on page 148)*

Overleaf: William Withering coaxes a secret cure for dropsy, or edema, from an old woman in Shropshire, England, in 1775. The physician identified the active herb as foxglove—the plant with bell-shaped flowers—which provides digitalis, a medicine for congestive heart failure.

141

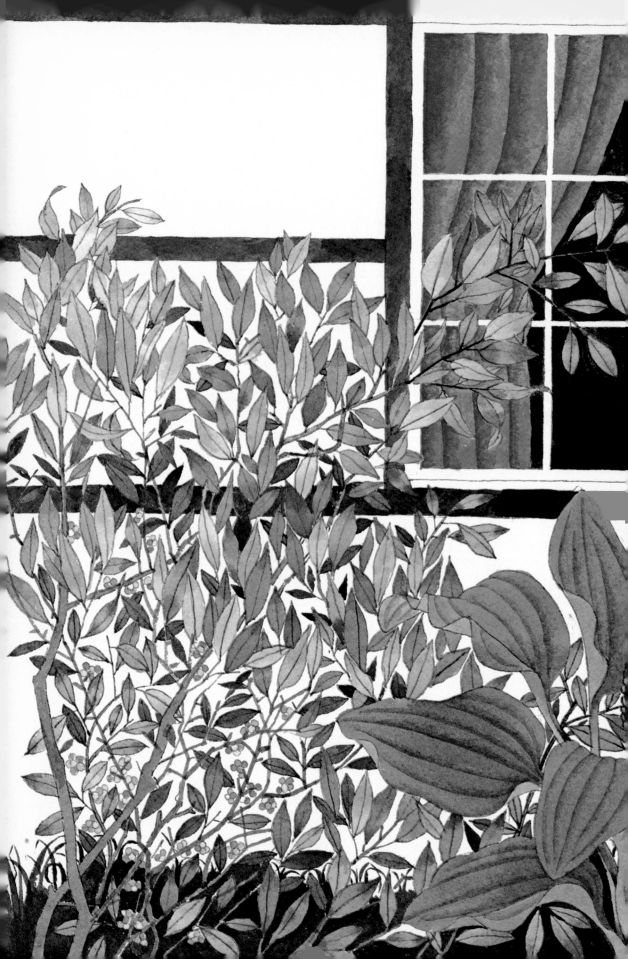

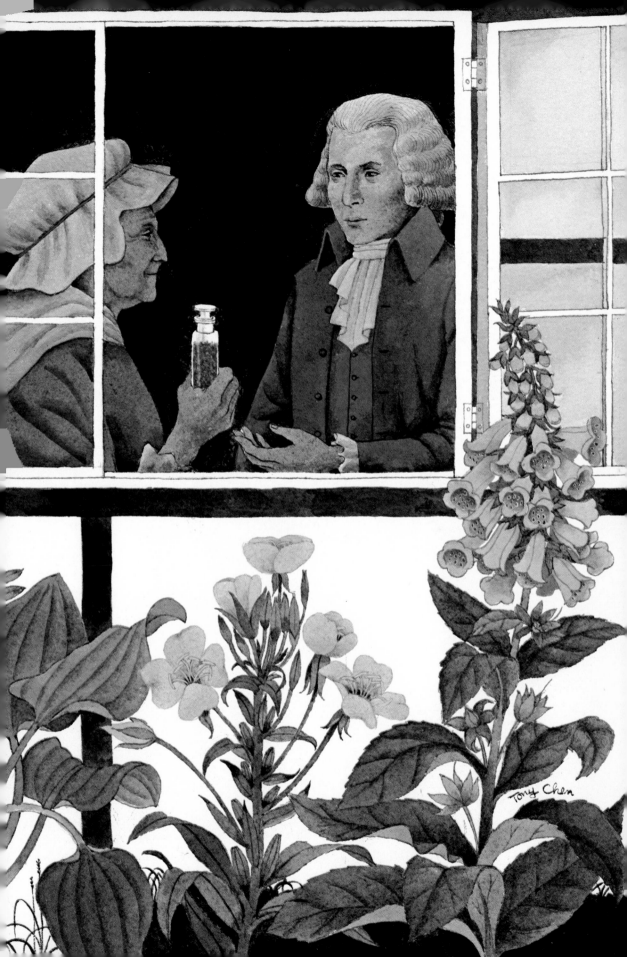

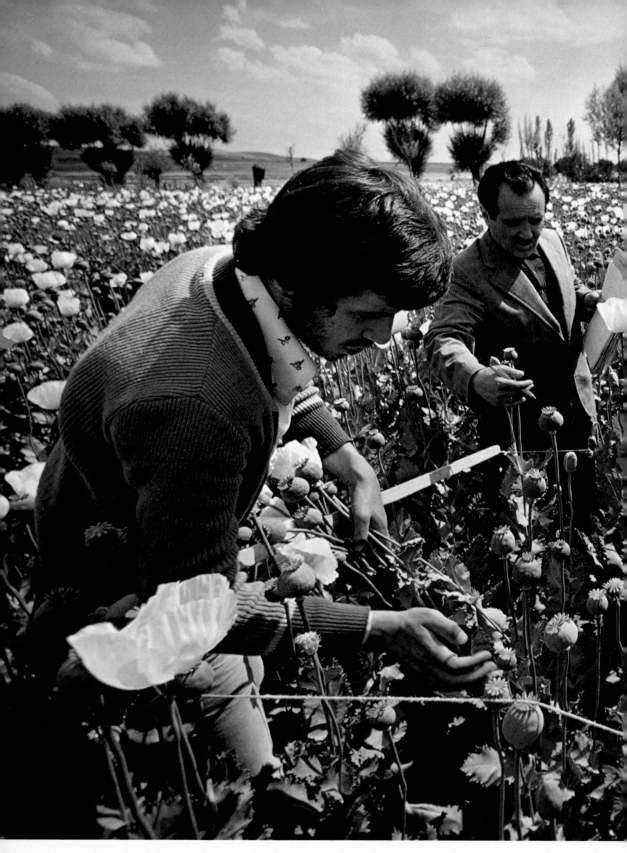

In spring, government officials measure fields in Turkey to control the yield of poppies,

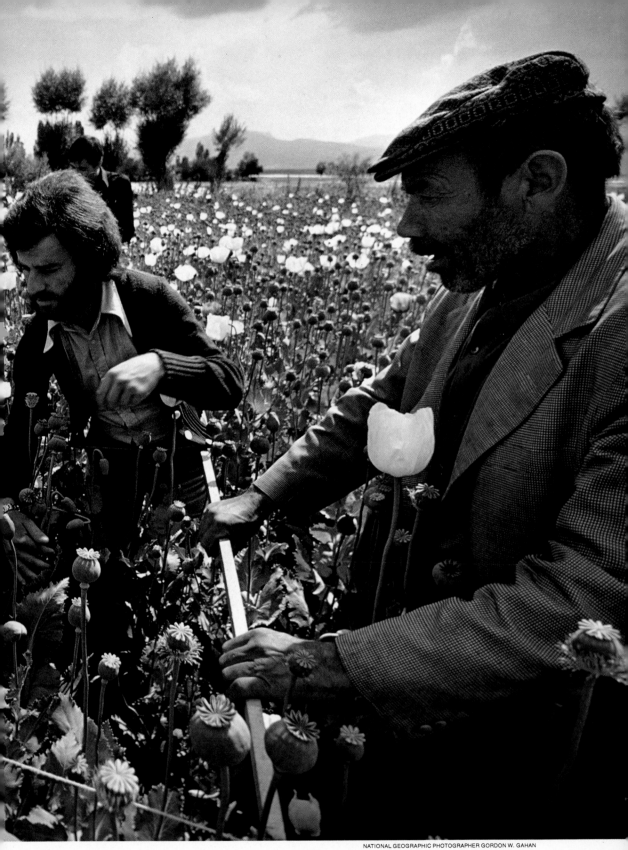

source of the painkillers morphine and codeine—and the illegal narcotic heroin.

Turkish farmers licensed to grow opium poppies pick the ripe seed heads, or capsules, in summer. A donkey (below, right) carries the capsules to town, where villagers remove the seeds for use in cooking. The remaining poppy straw—which contains the drug substance— goes to a government market (below) for subsequent sale to pharmaceutical firms. The resulting products, morphine and codeine, have proved invaluable in easing ailments— from coughs to terminal cancer.

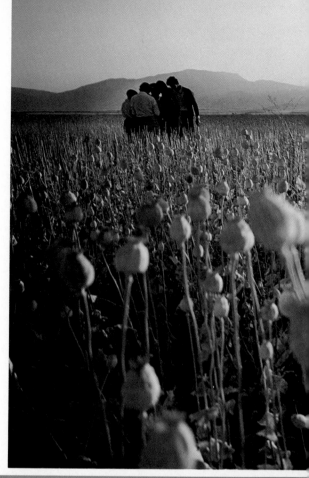

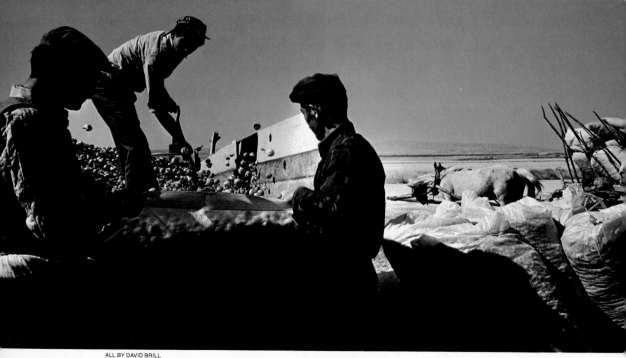

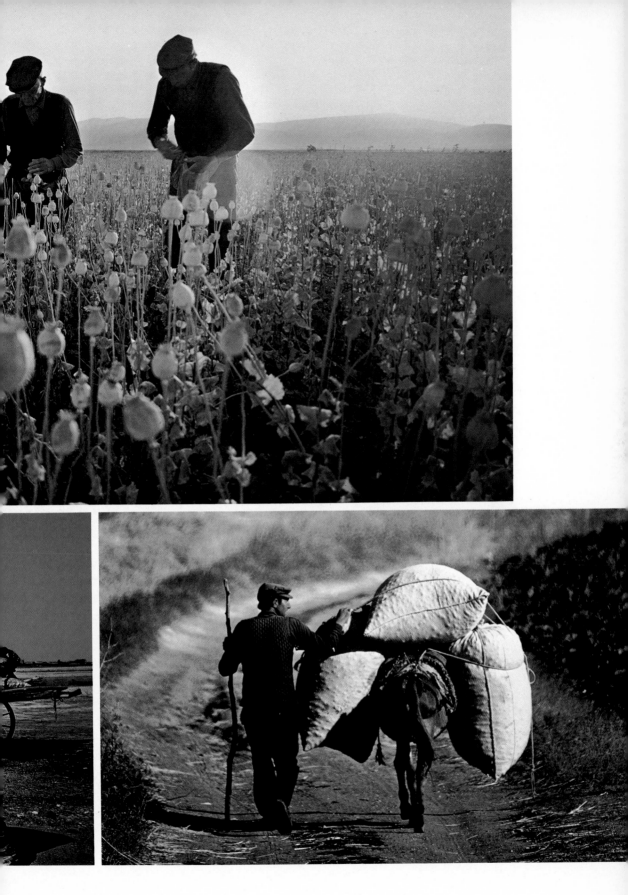

for two hours. Often compared to digitalis, it is useful in dropsical conditions, although, like squill, it may cause digestive disturbances.

No one knows how many more medicinal plants may hold glycosides to help the human heart. In an article published in *The Herbarist,* Dr. Richard Evans Schultes estimated that more than 400 kinds of cardioactive glycosides already have been isolated from the plant kingdom.

The animal kingdom also has something to contribute. The ancient Chinese made a medication for heart problems from dried skin of the common toad. This species is still listed as a cardiotonic by the Chinese, and Western scientists have confirmed the presence of its active substance.

There are times when medical practice seems to evoke the demonic arts of medieval witchcraft; in a scene from Shakespeare's *Macbeth,* a trio of witches chants, "Round about the cauldron go;/ In the poison'd entrails throw;/ . . . Fillet of a fenny snake,/ In the cauldron boil and bake;/ Eye of newt and toe of frog,/ Wool of bat and tongue of dog. . . ."

Today's physicians and surgeons are grateful for another exotic poison whose relaxing effect is opposite to that of heart stimulants. Its name is curare, and it provides active drugs that work with anesthetics and other medications to permit difficult operations and ease convulsive spasms from disease or accident.

In its native state, curare refers not to any one lethal compound, but to many related mixtures assembled by various South American tribes during centuries of hunting and warfare. It acts by paralyzing the victim, and kills by asphyxiation when paralysis reaches the respiratory muscles. Many Indians of the Amazon rain forests still concoct it, using tribal formulas. They smear it on arrows, blowgun darts, and spears to bring down game and, sometimes, enemies.

Of all jungle poisons, curare is perhaps the best known, partly because of its links with the dramas of exploration in the New World. Within half a century following the arrival of Columbus, Francisco de Orellana met Indians along the Amazon who introduced him to their curare-tipped arrows by killing one of his companions. Sir Walter Raleigh was horrified by curare in 1595 as he made his way up the Orinoco River in what is now Venezuela. The natives are "desperate people, and have the most strong poison on their arrowes," he wrote in his book, *The Discoverie of Guiana.* "Besides the mortalitie of the wound they make, the partie shot indureth the most insufferable torment in the world. . . ."

The talents and labors of many famous men joined to move curare from forest to laboratory and then to the operating room. In 1805, Germany's great geographer and traveler Alexander von Humboldt gave the scientific world its first reliable key to the poison's composition. He described a bitter, gummy mixture that he saw being boiled along the Upper

In the highlands of Peru, Eduardo Calderon—a curandero, or folk healer—picks a tree datura, a plant used for centuries to induce visions.

148

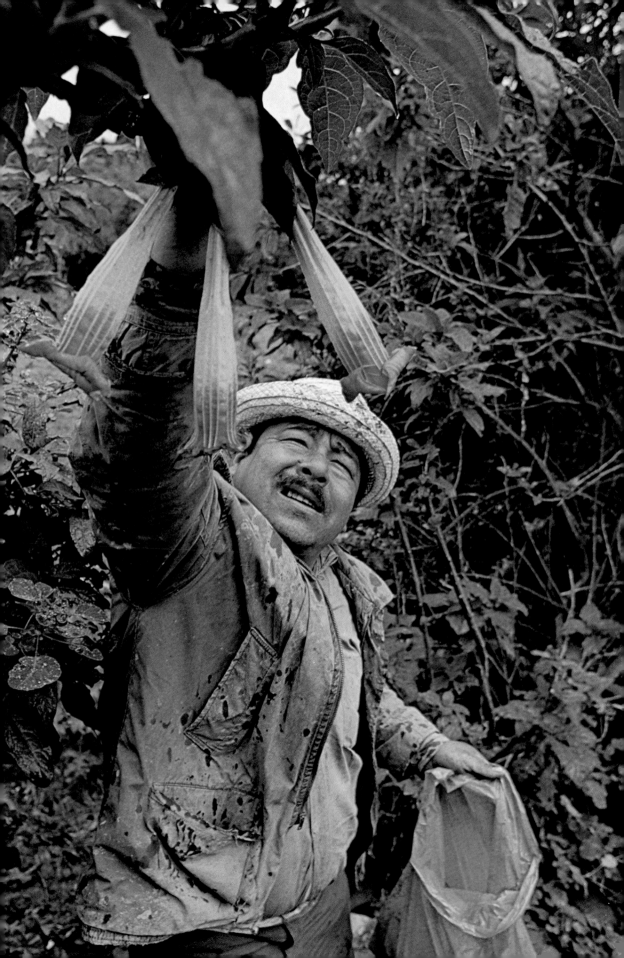

Entering a trance (below), Eduardo Calderon turns his attention inward. During a nightlong healing ceremony for a family (right), he uses herbal remedies (bottom, right) and curing rituals to lessen problems brought on by anxiety and social conflict. At center right, the curandero rubs a live guinea pig over another client. Eduardo will kill the animal and examine its organs to divine the cause of illness; he may recommend herbal cures or a visit to a physician. Eduardo, whose healing powers include the medicinal and the psychological, became a curandero in 1958 after a four-year apprenticeship, vowing to serve "without thought of gain. . .whatever the circumstances."

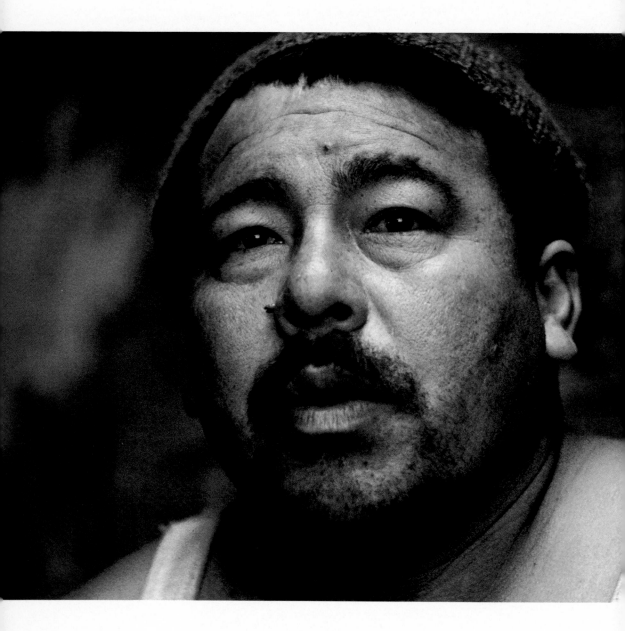

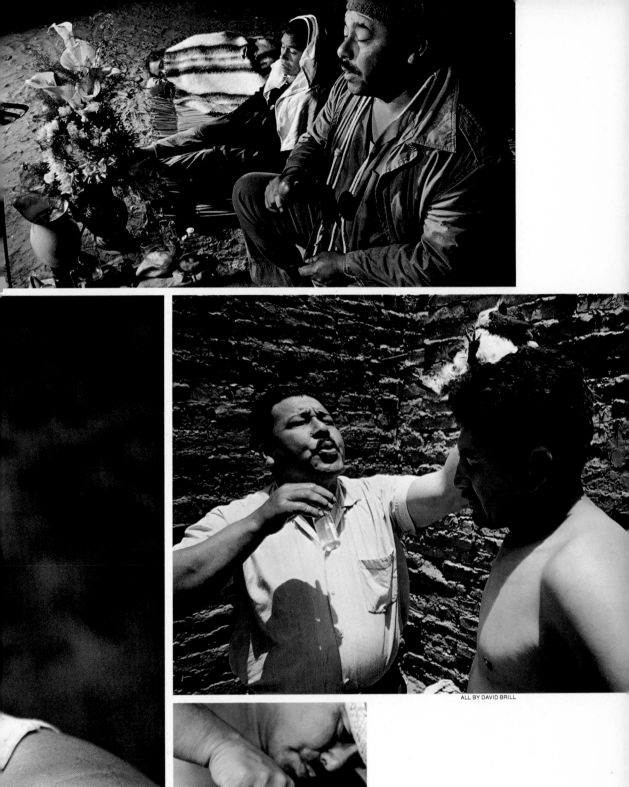

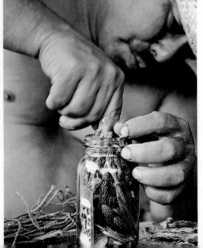

ALL BY DAVID BRILL

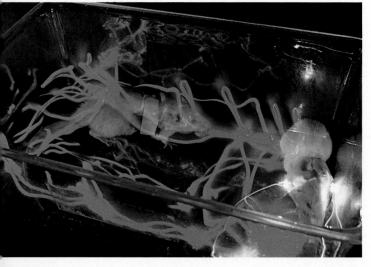

Movements of rats in an experiment concerning drug-induced hyperactivity show how high doses of cocaine affect behavior. The red light on a rat given cocaine illustrates — during a time exposure — compulsive repetitions of movement; the white light worn by an undrugged rat shows normal motion. Such studies may help reveal the functioning of nerve cells in abnormal behavior.

Orinoco as containing what was later judged to be the inner bark of a species of South American strychnine tree. About 1850, Claude Bernard of France, foremost physiologist of his time and an authority on the nervous system, discovered through experiments with frogs that the secret of the drug's paralysis lay in blocking impulses from the brain to the muscles.

Gradually, scientists isolated many muscle-relaxing alkaloids from curare. Beginning in the 1930's, these opened the way for both the natural and synthetic preparations that now exert their gentling influence on surgical and diagnostic procedures, and on the violent tensions of lockjaw, epilepsy, and other traumatic conditions.

But curare is another drug whose benefits are limited by the need to pinpoint the precarious balance between the dose that might save a patient and the one that might kill him. So, for many respiratory ailments, doctors turn to ephedrine, one of the oldest and most highly respected remedies in the world.

Ephedrine comes mainly from the stems of a low, unimpressive shrub that is native to northern and western China; it is known there as *Ma Huang*. Its bare, jointed, and brownish-green stems will never win any garden beauty prize, but its medical value against coughs and colds, asthma, hay fever, and other respiratory problems has been traditional for 5,000 years in China and elsewhere in the Orient.

The surprising fact about ephedrine, however, is the time that went by before the rest of the world took the drug, literally, to its chest. It was not until 1885 that a Japanese scientist even isolated the ephedrine alkaloid. Then 40 more years passed before an enterprising pair of physician-pharmacologists began to publish a series of papers on their experiments and studies that introduced the medical profession to the advantages of ephedrine drugs. Among the many conditions for which ephedrine and its synthetic derivatives are specifically prescribed are bronchial disorders, low blood pressure, and weak heart muscle.

Whether to use a natural or a synthetic drug is the choice, of course, of every physician, depending on the patient and the circumstances.

"For my own asthmatic patients I suggest an ephedra tea," said Dr. Andrew Weil, a research associate at the Botanical Museum of Harvard and a practicing physician in Tucson, Arizona; many people seek the dry climate of that region for relief from respiratory problems. "All those I've treated say they prefer ephedra tea to the isolated drug, because they get the same result without the side effects of a rapid heart beat and subsequent drained feeling. Apparently the secondary compounds in the whole plant modify the ephedrine when so taken."

It is never safe, however, to trust nature to modify. Some of the most dangerous plants of garden and field come dressed in beauty that lures the unwary. Back in the days of medicinal-plant discovery, primitive experimenters must often have paid with their lives to learn which plants could be swallowed without harm.

Archeologists have unearthed clay tablets from Babylonian and Assyrian ruins, proving that medical pioneers of these ancient civilizations fought illness with what we now know as deadly nightshade, henbane, and thorn apple, or jimsonweed. Modern physicians still regularly prescribe alkaloids obtained from these same three lethal plants.

Doctors call these natural alkaloids atropine, hyoscyamine, and scopolamine, and they are used to relieve muscular spasms of asthma and other respiratory or gastrointestinal ailments and to stimulate a flagging heart. One of the best known is deadly nightshade, or belladonna — beautiful lady — whose active substance was used by high-ranking women of the court in Renaissance Italy to enlarge the pupils of their eyes. It now helps ophthalmologists determine the proper lenses for eyeglasses.

Whether for vanity or for medicinal value, plants have been used for centuries. But at no time has interest been more acute than today as scientists search for natural products to attack the insidious disease of cancer. Medical researchers in the field of anticancer drugs find one of their most helpful leads in a series of articles published between 1967 and 1971 in the pharmacognosy journal *Lloydia*. These studies, which recount the folk use of tumor-treating plants since the earliest recorded times, were compiled by Dr. Jonathan L. Hartwell, who, until his retirement, headed the Natural Products Section of the Drug Development Branch of the National Cancer Institute near Washington.

It was there, Dr. Hartwell told me, that he first conceived of his massive research project. In his work as an organic chemist, he was isolating compounds from the white-flowered American herb mayapple, when he learned that Penobscot Indians of Maine had long employed this plant to cope with malignant and other growths. Further research turned up information that a resin from the dried roots of the same herb was listed in 1820

Snow-capped barrels of chemicals line a storage lot near a pilot plant of the Monsanto Research Corporation in Dayton, Ohio. The facility extracts maytansine—a possible anticancer drug—from the African shrub Maytenus buchananii. *Scientists at the University of Virginia and elsewhere worked for five years to isolate the compound and check its potential. Then Monsanto began producing the drug for clinical tests. A worker at the plant (below, left) shovels chipped bits of* Maytenus *into a mill. To produce just one ounce of maytansine requires more than 40 tons of stems. Below, a photomicrograph illuminated by polarized light reveals the drug's crystals. Two milligrams of maytansine—enough for a single dose—dust a thumbnail.*

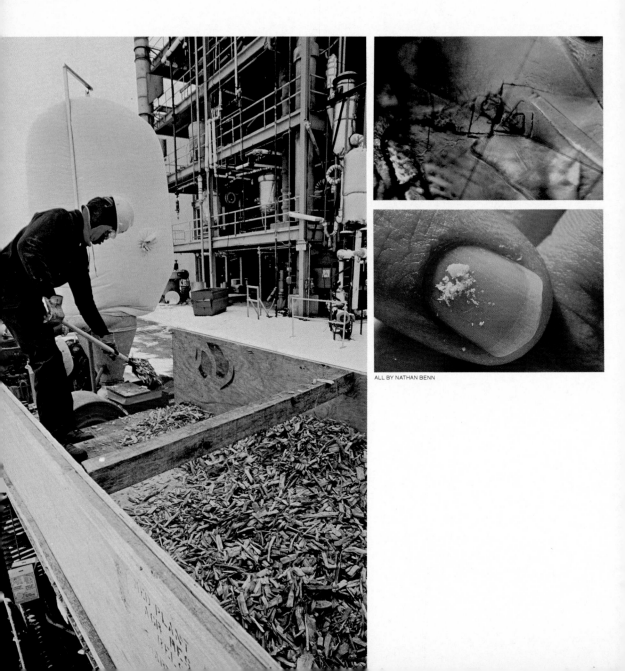

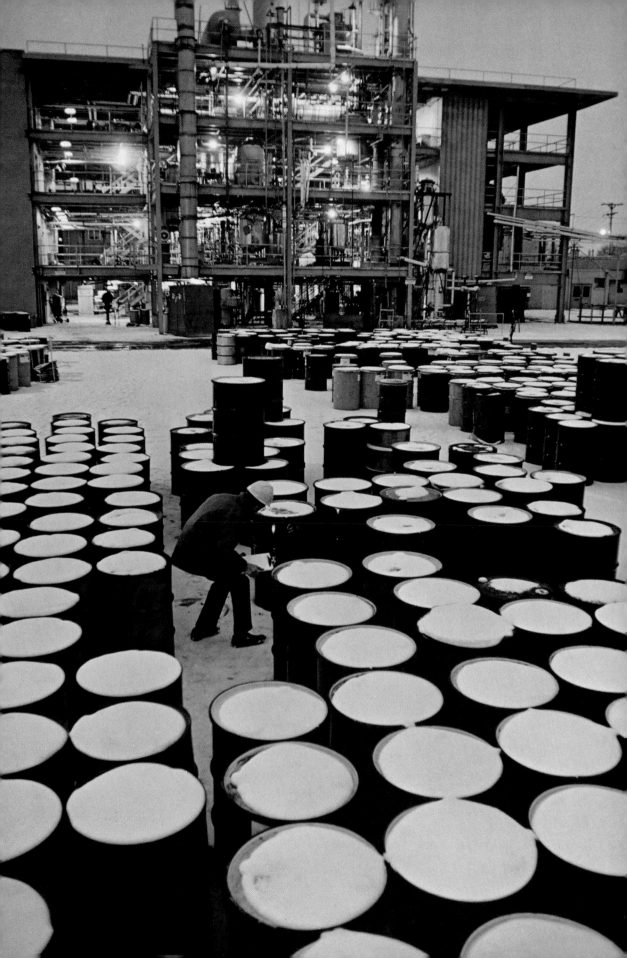

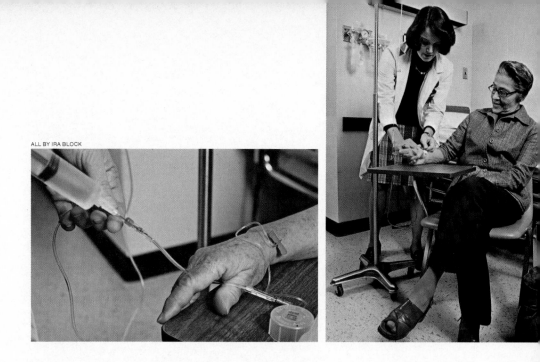

as a cathartic in the first *U. S. Pharmacopoeia,* and that physicians in Louisiana and Mississippi had prescribed it for cancer as recently as 1897. From this small beginning, Dr. Hartwell launched his survey that would eventually offer scientists valuable data on the correct botanical nature and past medical history of more than 3,000 plant species with potential anticancer properties.

As a postscript to the Hartwell catalog, it is instructive to note that species related to three plants described in it — periwinkle, mayapple, and *Maytenus* — now stand in the forefront of the fight against cancer.

Most important so far is the Madagascar periwinkle, related to the evergreen, ground-cover species found in North America. It already has contributed regularly prescribed drugs against leukemia and other forms of cancer. Mayapple and *Maytenus* have reached the stage of clinical trials against human cancer.

With its delicate white and rose petals, the Madagascar periwinkle seems an unlikely weapon to defeat a killer that is second only to heart disease in the United States. Yet even during the Roman Empire, folk healers were making salves and teas from another periwinkle plant to treat tumors, venomous bites, and dysentery.

In modern times, the reputation of the Madagascar periwinkle as a diabetes remedy led investigators to discover that its active principle worked, instead, against certain types of cancer. In the 1950's, two independent groups of researchers — Dr. Robert L. Noble and associates at Canada's University of Western Ontario, and Dr. Gordon H. Svoboda and co-workers at Eli Lilly — isolated from periwinkle leaves the first of the alkaloids that form the most effective drugs available for childhood leukemia and Hodgkin's disease, which attacks lymph glands, spleen, and liver.

How effective, I wondered, are vincristine and vinblastine, the

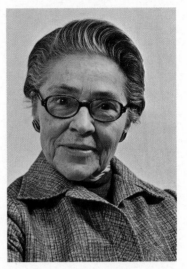

Caution and hope guide clinical tests of maytansine at the National Cancer Institute in Bethesda, Maryland. Enid Helfrich (right and opposite) and 41 other cancer patients have participated in the program. Since December 1976, she has taken the drug intravenously once every three weeks. It has initially stopped the spread of the disease. Dr. Bruce Chabner of the Institute says, "We are hopeful, but maytansine is still in the first phase of study. Of the compounds that reach clinical trial only one in 50,000 is ever marketed."

periwinkle drugs named for *Vinca,* the original botanical designation of the plant? According to Dr. Franco Muggia, Associate Director for Cancer Therapy Evaluation at the National Cancer Institute, the report is good. "A combination of vincristine with other drugs has brought remission for an average of five years in one half of the children suffering from leukemia," he said. "Doses of vincristine or vinblastine, each given with supporting medication, have resulted in ten-year remissions from advanced Hodgkin's disease in more than half of the cases."

There are still no synthetics to replace the raw leaves of the periwinkle. On my visit to the Lilly laboratories, I saw great bales of these leaves arriving from India, Madagascar, and other areas for processing into final liquid form as injectable doses. I learned how minute is the amount of active material obtained from each leaf. "It requires 12 to 15 tons of leaves to make just one ounce of vincristine sulfate," said pharmacognosist Svoboda. For his invention of intricate laboratory procedures to extract the tiny substance, he was presented the American Pharmaceutical Association's Research Achievement Award in Natural Products in 1963.

At the National Cancer Institute, I talked with Dr. John D. Douros, chief of the Natural Products Branch. I wanted to learn more about the role of plants and other natural products in the cancer therapy program conducted at the world's leading center for such research.

"When the hunt for anticancer drugs began at NCI in 1955, it was well known that plants contained potentially useful materials," Dr. Douros said. "In the first three years, 500 plant extracts were submitted for screening. The success of the *Vinca* drugs gave impetus to the work, and in 1960 a systematic effort was undertaken, with the cooperation of the Department of Agriculture, to obtain a worldwide variety of plants."

Since then, Dr. Douros explained, the Natural Products Branch has

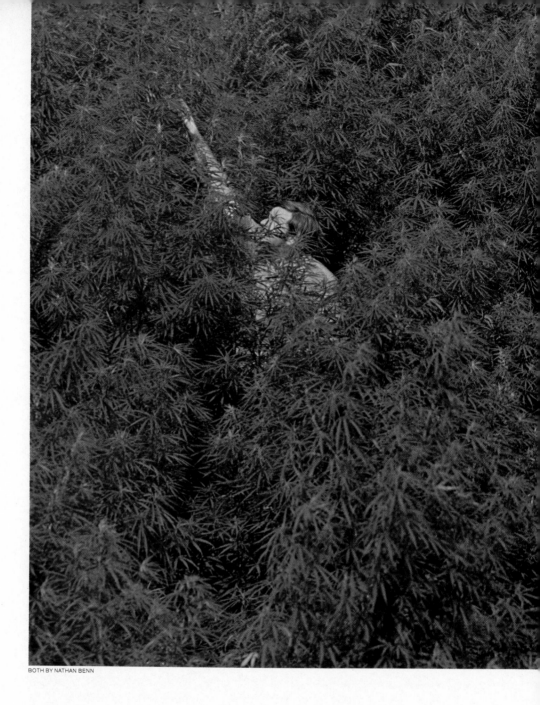

Thick, leafy marijuana plants nearly obscure a worker at the Research Institute of Pharmaceutical Sciences in Oxford, Mississippi. On this 5.6-acre tract, the Institute grows all the marijuana used in government-sponsored research. At right, smoke shrouds a field hand as he burns parts of the plant not needed in scientific investigation. Since 1967, the government has spent about 20 million dollars on the study of marijuana. Preliminary findings show the drug may prove effective against glaucoma and asthma, and control such side effects as nausea in cancer treatment.

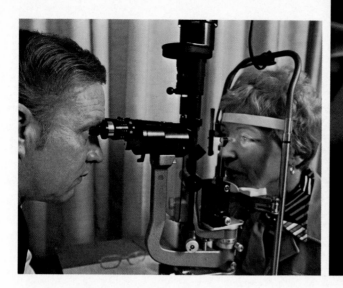

maintained contracts for the regular collection of thousands of species of plants. The crude samples are gathered largely at random and put through a series of rigorous tests, beginning at one of the Institute's laboratory facilities. There, plants that yield extracts showing antitumor activity against laboratory cultures and animals are singled out to be re-collected in larger quantities.

If extracts from these roots and barks and fruits continue to confirm activity, they are sent to other research laboratories for the purification and isolation of compounds that account for such activity. In turn, these compounds undergo a series of further trials in which a safe dosage is set for humans through tests on dogs and monkeys.

Finally comes the moment of truth for drugs that have made it through all preliminary stages. NCI is now ready to present them for review to clinical cancer specialists who meet several times a year at the Institute. They will administer selected compounds to specific patients for treatment and observation.

This is the point that mayapple and *Maytenus,* the most promising plants since the Madagascar periwinkle, have reached today.

From the dried roots of mayapple, the herb that introduced Dr. Hartwell to cancer folklore, have come derivatives called podophyllotoxins. "These compounds," says Dr. Muggia, "have shown strong activity against leukemias and lymph tumors, and, to some degree, against brain, bladder, and lung tumors."

Maytenus, a plant that grows as a flowering vinelike shrub throughout tropical Africa, is one of the latest additions to anticancer research. It was first discovered in Ethiopia in 1962 as part of a random collection for the NCI program. Then, in the 1970's, Dr. Robert E. Perdue, Jr., who heads the Department of Agriculture's Medicinal Plant Resources Laboratory at

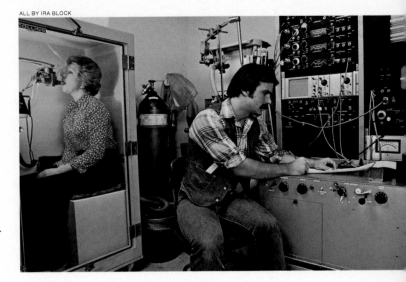

Studies at a Los Angeles school of medicine point to marijuana's potential as a useful drug. With an applanation tonometer (far left), a researcher examines a woman's cornea and measures pressure inside her eye. (left). Marijuana may aid glaucoma by reducing intraocular pressure. The drug also dilates bronchial tubes, making breathing easier for asthmatics. A body plethysmograph (right) records dilation in a woman's bronchial tubes.

Beltsville, Maryland, found a more productive species in the Shimba Hills of Kenya. He has now collected some 60,000 pounds of this shrub.

Meantime, a group of chemists, directed by the late Dr. S. Morris Kupchan at the University of Virginia in Charlottesville, had isolated maytansine, the plant's chief anticancer agent. They then determined its structure in a five-year project deemed extraordinary in the field.

"It is highly active against animal tumors and yet appears to be relatively nontoxic," Dr. Kupchan said of the compound. "It may be very useful in treating human cancers."

In a report delivered in May 1977 at the annual meeting of the American Association for Cancer Research, Dr. Bruce Chabner of the National Cancer Institute summed up the plant's potential in the results of early tests conducted on 35 adults and 7 children.

"Of the patients treated so far," he said, "three give evidence of responding to the drug. There has been a decrease in the tumor volume in a case each of childhood leukemia, ovarian cancer, and a malignancy of the lymph node system. We consider the results sufficiently promising to continue trials with specific types of cancer over the next several years."

After 17 years of collecting, developing, and testing plants, the NCI program may be "only now reaching the point of maximum return in terms of materials being prepared for clinical trial," said Dr. Saul A. Schepartz, deputy director of the program.

Especially significant to those who deal with natural products, I found, is the estimate that twice as many of these substances are in advanced stages of clinical testing today as there were a few years ago. "Right now," Dr. Douros said, "about 60 percent of the drugs are still synthetic, but natural compounds from microorganisms, as well as those from the higher plants, are taking an ever larger part."

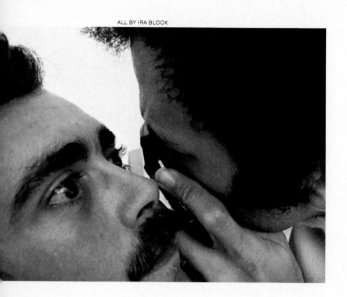

Suffering from glaucoma, Robert Randall of Washington, D. C., smokes a marijuana cigarette from an official Federal Government packet to relieve pressure in his eyes. Randall smokes as many as eight such cigarettes each day as part of a government-licensed study administered by Dr. John Merritt of Howard University. Dr. Merritt hopes to determine the drug's impact on glaucoma and test a marijuana-based eye drop to treat it. He examines Randall (left) each week and prescribes an exact dosage.

As the work goes on, drug seekers are collecting plants to heal not only the ravaged body. In the laboratory and in the wild, scientists concerned with problems of the mind are also looking for hallucinogenic and narcotic compounds. Such compounds may help psychotic patients by providing comparisons between induced and abnormal conditions.

This interest in natural drugs that alter mind and mood is relatively new to Western science. "In general our medical forebears accepted quite readily the native remedies that would heal a wound or reduce a fever," said Dr. Nathan S. Kline, director of the Rockland Research Institute in Orangeburg, New York, and a leading advocate of drug therapy for the mentally disturbed. "They balked, however, when confronted with anything that seemed to touch the mind or spirit."

The first such psychotropic, or mind-affecting, drug to gain wide Western acceptance came from the root of *Rauwolfia serpentina*. A climbing shrub native to India and neighboring countries, it was named for Leonhard Rauwolf, a 16th-century botanist. Western psychiatrists, however, were thousands of years behind the medicine men of India in recognizing the remarkable qualities of this plant. Ancient Sanskrit and other Hindu manuscripts had mentioned it among useful medicinal herbs, and Indian folk healers continued through the centuries to consider it a panacea for everything from venomous bites to cholera. Of even greater significance, *Rauwolfia* was especially popular as a source of soothing medications and a cure for "moon madness," or lunacy—a striking hint of its future use in Western medicine.

Rauwolfia got its modern start in the early 1950's as the first tranquilizer in Western therapy. Before that time, interest in the plant's chemical nature had been largely confined to scientific circles in India. The first notable contribution to the subject appeared in 1931, with the publication in

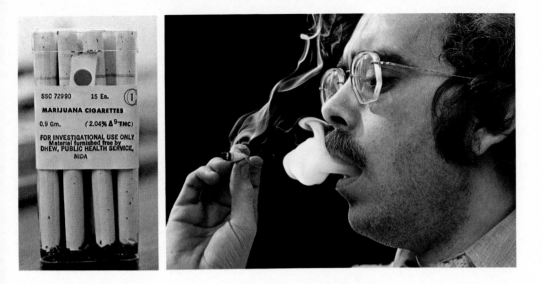

the *Journal of the Indian Chemical Society* of a report by two Indian research chemists who had isolated five new alkaloids from crude *Rauwolfia* roots. At about the same time, two Indian physicians announced that they, too, had isolated similar alkaloids, and that patients treated with the whole powdered root had gained relief from high blood pressure, insomnia, and certain forms of insanity.

There the matter rested until increasing reports from the East on *Rauwolfia*'s value in controlling high blood pressure led Western scientists to take note. In 1952, chemists of a Swiss pharmaceutical company isolated the root's most effective alkaloid, reserpine, which was then marketed under the name of Serpasil.

Then, in 1954, came an event that gave worldwide publicity to *Rauwolfia* as a treatment for mental illness. As Dr. Kline tells the story in his book, *From Sad to Glad,* it was through "chance circumstances" that he decided to hold a series of cautious trials with both the *Rauwolfia* plant and its new drug, using patients at the Rockland State Hospital. He first selected a few schizophrenic and manic-depressive patients, then followed with 700 others in a broad range of cases.

The rest is history. So spectacular were the effects of reserpine in reducing the tensions of moderately disturbed patients and calming the violence of more seriously ill ones, that enthusiastic proponents predicted that mental institutions would soon be emptied of patients. Though *Rauwolfia* failed to live up to such extravagant hopes, and other drugs have since replaced it in treating most cases of mental illness, reserpine's early use allowed many thousands of once hopeless hospital patients to return to their homes and lead normal, or nearly normal, lives.

Moreover, dozens of reserpine-like compounds, natural and synthetic, have now become the world's most widely prescribed drugs for high

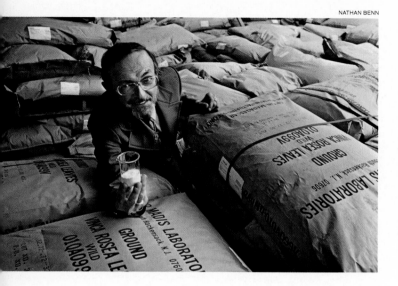

Surrounded by sacks of Madagascar periwinkle leaves, Dr. Gordon Svoboda of Eli Lilly holds a beaker of vincristine sulfate. Some 12 to 15 tons of the leaf yield just one ounce of the drug. Vincristine, taken with other drugs, has a cure rate of almost 50 percent for childhood leukemia over a period of five years. "It's the best answer we have so far," says Dr. Svoboda.

blood pressure, supporting an industry involving billions of dollars a year.

Like the *Vinca* saga, the *Rauwolfia* success story has had far-reaching consequences. One result was to stimulate a global search for other mind-affecting drugs. In the United States, the drive helped push a bill through Congress to establish the National Institute of Mental Health, and to set up within it a psychopharmacology section. This section would obtain such drugs by awarding grants to qualified professionals for field and laboratory work.

To the new breed of mind researchers, three of the most bizarre psychoactive plants were already at hand in the 1950's, because of the intellectual curiosity and dedicated labors of Harvard's Richard Evans Schultes, often called "dean of the plant hunters."

His fascination with plant drugs that change perception and behavior began with his first field expedition to investigate the magical and medicinal use of the peyote cactus by the Kiowa Indians of Oklahoma. At that time, he became one of the few outsiders ever to witness the peyote rites practiced by the widespread and now generally legalized Indian faith, the Native American Church.

On subsequent travels in Mexico, after reading accounts of Spanish chroniclers, he rediscovered and botanically identified two hallucinogenic plants that, together with peyote, had been sacred to the Aztecs. These plants were a morning glory vine called *ololiuqui* and a mushroom called *teonanacatl,* known as "flesh of the gods" to the Indians, but as an object of loathing to disapproving Spaniards.

Later, during his many years in the Amazon Basin, Dr. Schultes found still other psychoactive plants used by aboriginal tribes of Colombia, Brazil, and Venezuela to seek the supernatural world through wildly intoxicating religious and curing ceremonies. Among the most important of these are various species of a tree of the *Virola* genus, a member of the nutmeg family. From the blood-red resin of its inner bark, Indians make a potent hallucinogenic snuff—from which chemists have obtained a number of psychedelic compounds.

Curiously, however, as the modern science of drug therapy has advanced over the past quarter century, the old Aztec mind benders have led all such substances in psychiatric research. From them have come dozens of alkaloids to probe the workings of abnormal minds.

To appreciate the nature of this research, one must understand how hallucinogens act on the central nervous system. Mescaline, from the dried tops of peyote, causes visions in color and shape that may be terrifying or delightful. Similar sensations follow intoxication by lysergic acid amide—from the seeds of certain species of morning glories—or by psilocybin from Mexico's "magic mushrooms."

Added to the ancient hallucinogens in 1938 was another psychoactive drug, discovered by the Swiss chemist Albert Hofmann, who called it LSD—lysergic acid diethylamide. Derived synthetically from ergot, a common fungus growth on rye, LSD turned out to be chemically related to the other three, but 20 times more potent than the most powerful one.

At the National Institute of Mental Health, I asked about these and other drugs that are being tested in the research laboratories and used in the hospital there for selected cases of mental illness.

"At one time or another, we have used derivatives of peyote, mushrooms, and ergot, as well as reserpine, cocaine, and the active ingredient of marijuana," said Dr. Frederick K. Goodwin, chief of the Institute's Clinical Psychobiology Branch. "They served in studies to evaluate the mental and physical effects of such drugs in normal control and in patients with manic-depressive and schizophrenic illnesses.

"But natural products now play a minor role," he continued, "since they've been replaced generally by more specific-acting synthetics. The only major exception of a natural drug employed extensively here and elsewhere is lithium carbonate, a simple salt from the alkali metal group. It has proved to be quite successful in treating manic-depressive psychoses, and is the major breakthrough of this decade.

"We should not forget, however," Dr. Goodwin said, "the significance of natural products in the original observations that led to scientific research on the relation of brain chemistry to psychiatric disturbances. In my opinion, the chief advances in psychiatry in the last 25 or 30 years have been in the field of psychopharmacology. In fact, I would not be surprised at all to see some natural discovery become the basis for a whole new class of drugs."

Overleaf: At a crowded bazaar in Patna, India, physicians Salimuzzaman and Rafat Siddiqui purchase Rauwolfia *root in 1931. Their early studies of the root led to the eventual isolation of reserpine, the first tranquilizer.*

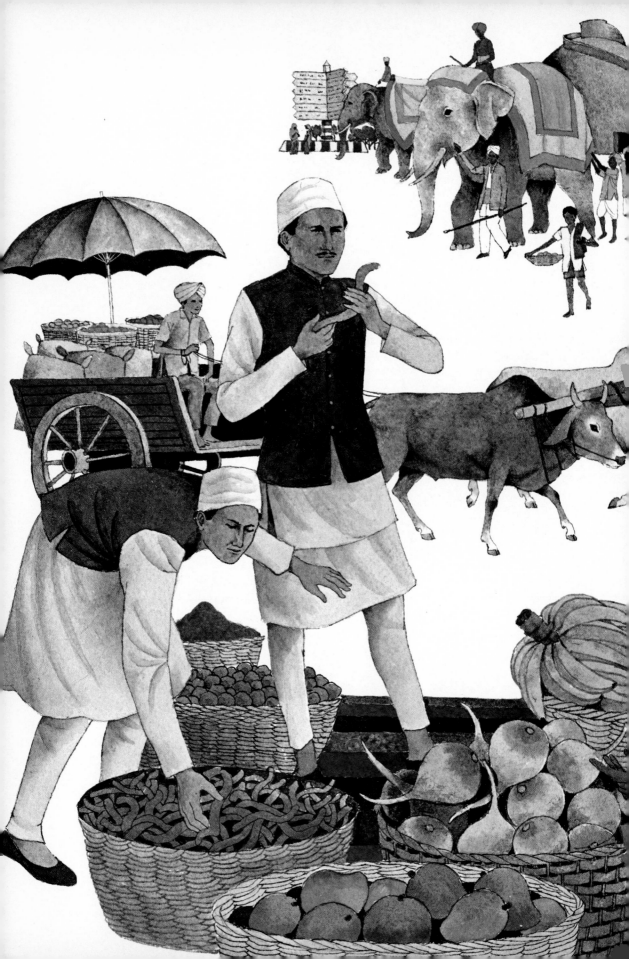

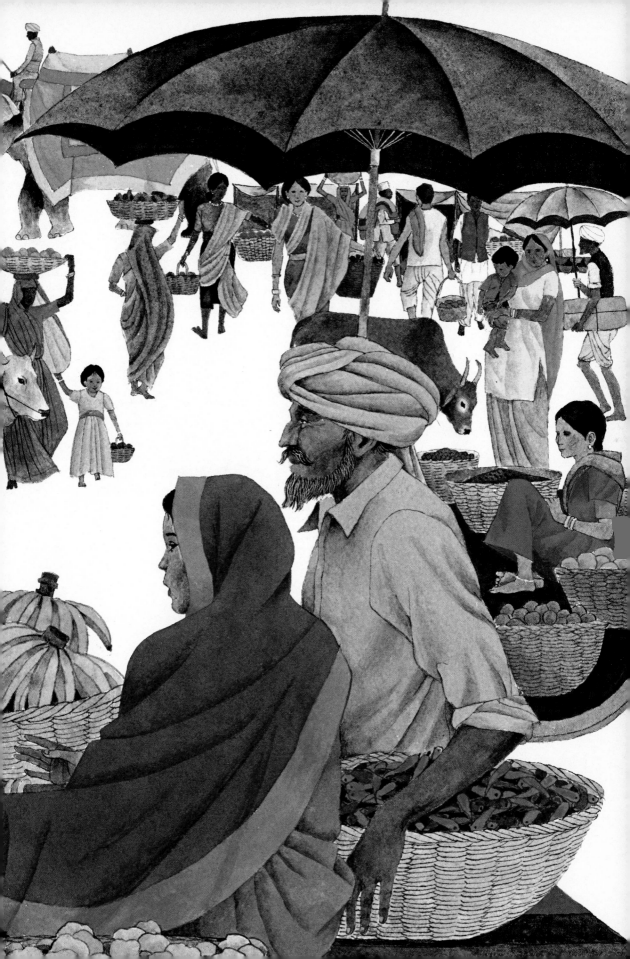

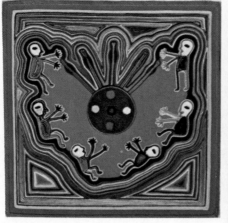

Ceremonial fire casts flickering light on Huichol Indians in Mexico. In an ancient ritual to communicate with their deities, they eat peyote—a potent hallucinogen—which they had dug earlier (below). A colorful yarn painting depicts the finding of peyote. Scientists consider the plant a valuable tool in the study of mental illness.

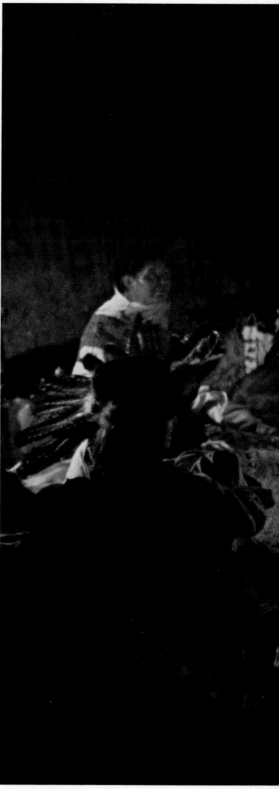

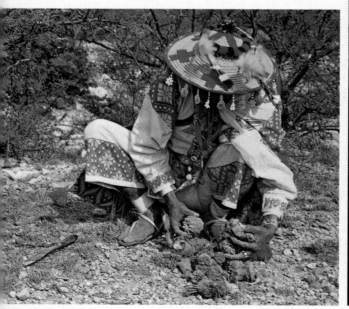

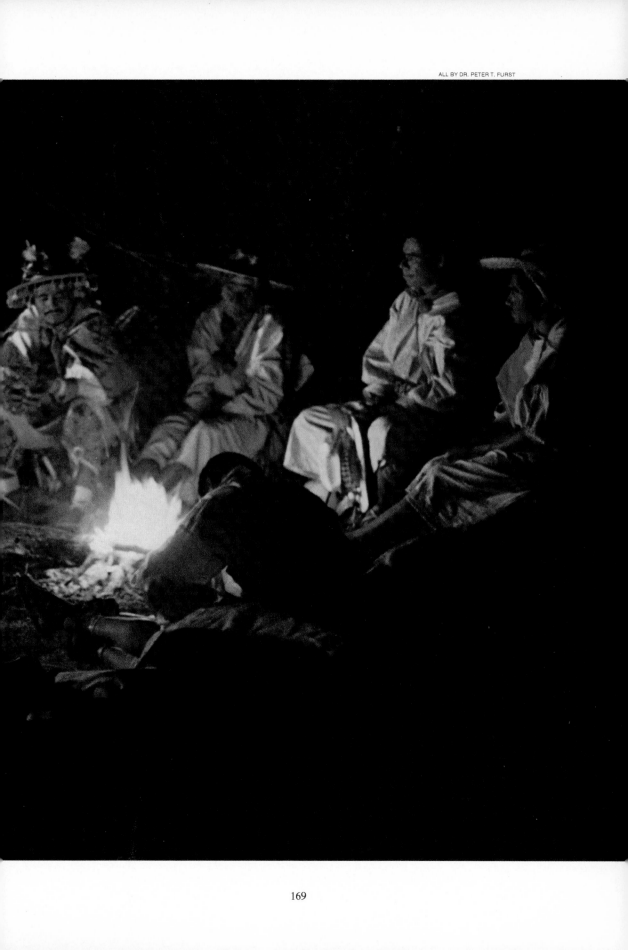

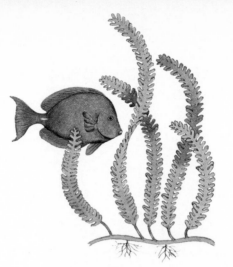

In Pursuit
of Health

"THE HAZARDS IN THIS JOB come not so much from big, fierce-looking creatures like sharks and barracudas as from two-inch blobs of jelly," said Ray Granade, raising his voice above the din of our motorboat.

"I found that out when I was diving near the shore over there to collect surgeonfish. Suddenly I felt a pain in my shoulder just like a whiplash. I had tangled with a jellyfish called a sea wasp. The sting of a sea wasp has been known to kill some people by drowning, after first causing shock. It certainly stunned me for the moment, and several days passed before I got over the painful burning."

Ray's excruciating experience with the jellyfish provided a graphic illustration of the value of undersea products to medicine, for a serum that alleviates the pain of an attack has been developed from the pure toxin of the sea wasp itself. The Australian Serum Laboratory in Sydney produces the remedy from a local species of the sea wasp.

I had joined Ray Granade on my first trip to the sounds and inlets of the British Virgin Islands in the Caribbean Sea. I was investigating the research at a field station on Virgin Gorda; work there is directed by Dr. Norman J. Doorenbos, professor of pharmacognosy at the University of

Reaching inside an oxygen-free chamber, Dr. Fred Counter of Eli Lilly dilutes an antibiotic for testing. Scientists today have broadened the search for new natural drugs to include plants and animals from the sea.

CAULERPA AND SURGEONFISH (ABOVE)

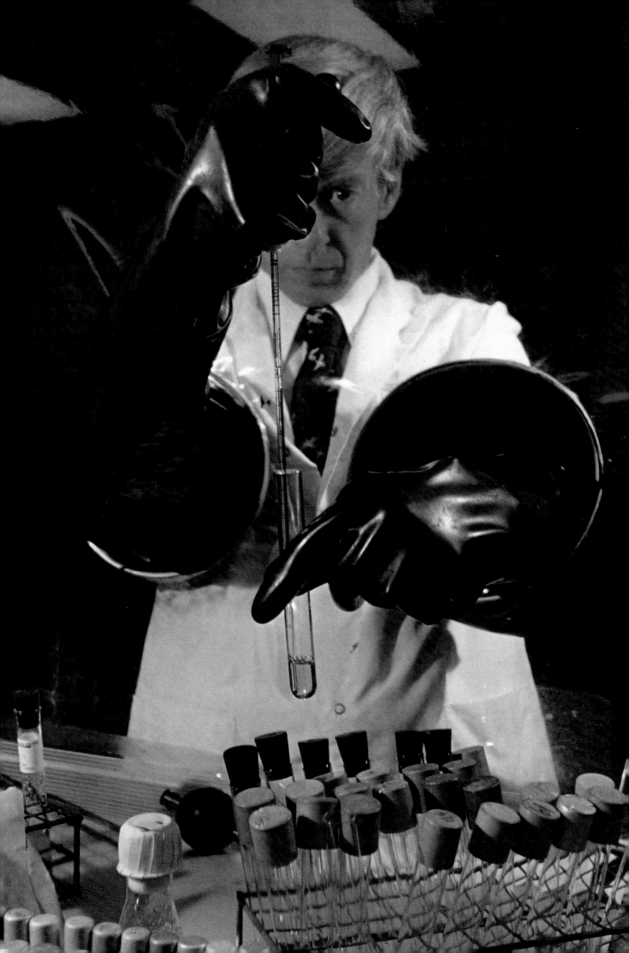

Mississippi. Ray is a graduate student at "Ole Miss" and one of a group of young pharmacognosists engaged in diving and scientific studies there.

An intense man with unruly, sun-bleached hair, Ray is active in many phases of the search for biochemical products from the sea. "We have to start with nature in looking for new compounds," he told me, "because that's where we get the original substances we need to extract and identify for further pharmacological research.

"The sea offers a promising source of drugs because many of the organisms that live in this environment have developed strongly toxic defense substances through the long struggle for survival against lethal enemies. Some of these substances may result in useful medications that have not been discovered in land organisms, or may replace those that have lost their potency as a result of bacterial resistance.

"How do we know what to look for in these waters? First," he said, "we learn from the local people which fish or plants are considered most poisonous, and where recent outbreaks of illness from eating them or being in contact with them have occurred. Then we collect samples in the suspect waters. In general, the more toxic the sea life, the better our chances of discovering a potentially active material."

On my maiden voyage into the techniques of fishing for medicine, I began to understand what research divers go through to catch their specimens. Early one morning, I watched Ray and his colleagues stow heavy gear on the deck of the *Reef Sampler,* our 34-foot motored transport. With them they brought the usual diving equipment of snorkels, inflated vests, belt weights to overcome the water's buoyancy, insulated wet suits, and compressed-air tanks for deep dives.

Then came the tools—long knives to slash tangled vegetation, small knives and scissors to snip out tissue from corals, and, for larger game, spear guns measuring six feet long.

The weather that day was hardly a vacationer's dream of balmy Caribbean climes and sunny beaches. So strong were the winds and so rough the waves that Ray passed up the plan to collect specimens along a line of submerged reefs in open water. Instead we rolled and pitched, in driving rain, to anchor in a more sheltered area.

One by one, the divers jumped in. Swimming at first, their orange-tipped snorkels popping up here and there above the whitecaps, they finally disappeared into depths of some 60 feet. An hour of silence followed. When they finally resurfaced, I was as eager as a child to see what they had brought. "We took samples of plant and animal life," said Ray, displaying plastic test tubes and nylon sacks with cuttings. "This plant is *Caulerpa,* a bright green alga that can grow very deep. Toxic species of it have been found in the Pacific. The rest are animals—sponges and soft corals, or gorgonians. We need only tiny amounts like this, since we get millions of organisms from a single gram of material. Also, if we snip out a small sample, it doesn't damage the animal.

"Sponges are particularly interesting to us," he said, "because there are perhaps more species of bacteria and other organisms in these animals than can be found anywhere else. To illustrate their potential value, three compounds of a Caribbean sponge served as models for a synthetic drug marketed as Cytosar. It's used against acute leukemia."

As a landlubber, I was fascinated by the minute gorgonians scooped out of their finger-shaped skeletons. Marine scientists consider these pin-head-size blobs of tissue highly promising as producers of antibiotic and other therapeutic agents. Some extracts have shown activity in stimulating muscular action, inducing labor, and in controlling fertility.

Following subsequent dives with the drug hunters off Eustatia, Prickly Pear, and Salt islands, we returned to port on Virgin Gorda bearing bags filled with other specimens: sea cucumber, sea urchin, sea hare—a kind of mollusk—goatfish, and surgeonfish.

Many of these creatures, as well as other kinds of underwater Caribbean species, may hold new compounds to treat heart and respiratory conditions, gastrointestinal troubles, tumors, or other ills. Sea cucumbers yield toxic chemical compounds called holothurins, now being studied for their effect on the nervous system and for their activity against cancer. Toxins from goatfish have been found to produce hallucinations, suggesting potential psychiatric applications. And the queen conch contains substances which appear to inhibit diseases such as polio and influenza.

In addition to their search for other new medications, the young scientists of Virgin Gorda are pursuing bacterial clues to the long-mysterious origin of a tropical fish poisoning known as ciguatera. A major health problem of the Caribbean, ciguatera may come from eating contaminated fish, especially such large varieties as barracuda, kingfish, and horse-eye jack. In moderate cases, the symptoms resemble those of a gastrointestinal attack, plus a numbness or tingling sensation around the mouth and in the limbs. Severe cases, however, may bring convulsions, coma, and death by respiratory paralysis.

"This is our laboratory, where we hope to learn about the nature and origin of ciguatera," said Ray, as we entered a small frame building lined with equipment. "We use mostly surgeonfish for our experiments because they are common in contaminated areas. Mounting evidence suggests that the disease may be caused by toxins from some microorganism, or perhaps from many species of microorganisms found in the intestinal tracts of such plant-eating fish.

"In other words, a surgeonfish may ingest toxic bacteria along with the algae it eats. In turn the contaminated surgeonfish may be consumed by a barracuda, which then also becomes toxic. If we can isolate the bacteria from toxic fish, and then establish the specific nature of the toxicity, medicinal chemists should be able eventually to produce a remedy a physician could prescribe."

Before leaving Virgin Gorda, I heard of a treatment for ciguatera that was old there long before laboratory analysis of folk medicines was ever developed. A tea brewed from the leaves of the buttonwood bush, say the islanders, brings rapid relief from the disease's symptoms, including the intense itching that often occurs.

"Does the tea really work?" I asked Dr. Doorenbos, who spends several months a year on his Caribbean project.

"The local people believe it does," he answered. "We'll test this remedy with laboratory animals as soon as we have enough of the ciguatera toxin to begin such studies. Ray Granade has already found bacteria in surgeonfish which produce toxins that resemble ciguatera. If these toxins are proven to be ciguatera, we can prepare large quantities of the scarce toxin for further research. We've discovered that the bacteria will produce toxins when grown in our laboratory on the Mississippi campus. Now it may be possible to develop a test to determine if a reef fish is toxic before it is eaten. If so, the discovery would help many people, since ciguatera is a problem throughout the world."

To find out what's new at one of the first American colleges of pharmacy to cast its nets for drugs from the sea, I flew north from the Caribbean to the University of Rhode Island at Kingston.

"We've by no means dropped our search for biomedical compounds from land plants and animals," said Dr. Heber W. Youngken, Jr., professor of pharmacognosy at the College of Pharmacy and an authority on both terrestrial and marine subjects. "But we're now devoting our energies chiefly to meeting the challenge of finding drugs underwater. This interest has been part of the university curriculum since 1964. Then in 1967 we joined the National Sea Grant Program, which provides funds to certain universities for wide-ranging marine studies.

"At present, our marine research concerns a green seaweed and several red ones which may provide anticancer compounds. We are also investigating several other kinds of algae that play a part in the periodic attacks of the red tide. Dr. Yuzuru Shimizu, professor of pharmacognosy here, is directing the red tide studies. He's going out this afternoon on a collecting trip with some of his students. He'll be glad to take you along."

At Beaver Tail Point on the tip of Conanicut Island, we parked our cars and scrambled down a steep incline. We then hopped across great craggy rocks all the way to the water's edge.

There, with the outgoing tide foaming at our feet, Dr. Shimizu and his students rolled up their pants legs and *(Continued on page 184)*

Fishing for medicine: In the Caribbean Sea off Virgin Gorda, marine pharmacognosists raise a fish trap with specimens for medicinal research. At the University of Mississippi's field station on the island, they screen a variety of undersea organisms that may yield new drug compounds.

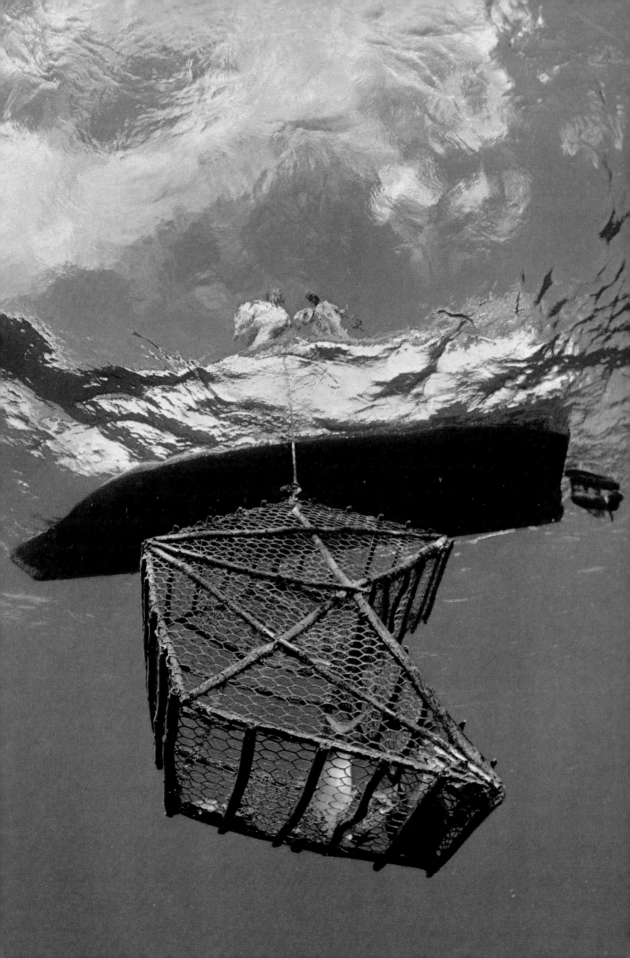

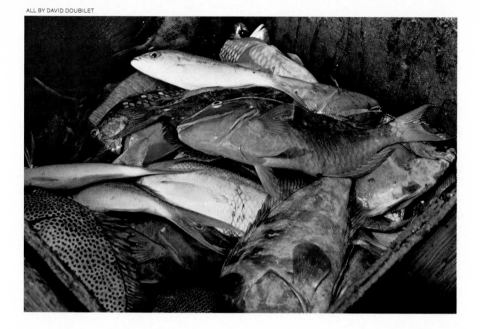

Buttonwood bush tea simmers over a fire on a Virgin Gorda beach. Islanders drink the bitter brew to relieve symptoms of a tropical fish poisoning known as ciguatera—a major health problem in many parts of the Caribbean. Eating contaminated fish may cause the disease, and a typical local catch (above) might contain some toxic specimens. Frank Harrigan uses the tea remedy when he suffers from ciguatera. After picking fresh buttonwood leaves (below), he boils and strains the mixture, then sips the dark tea.

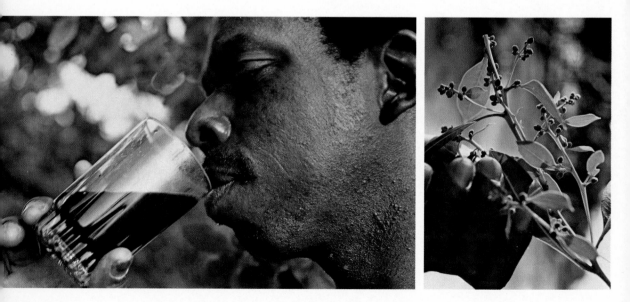

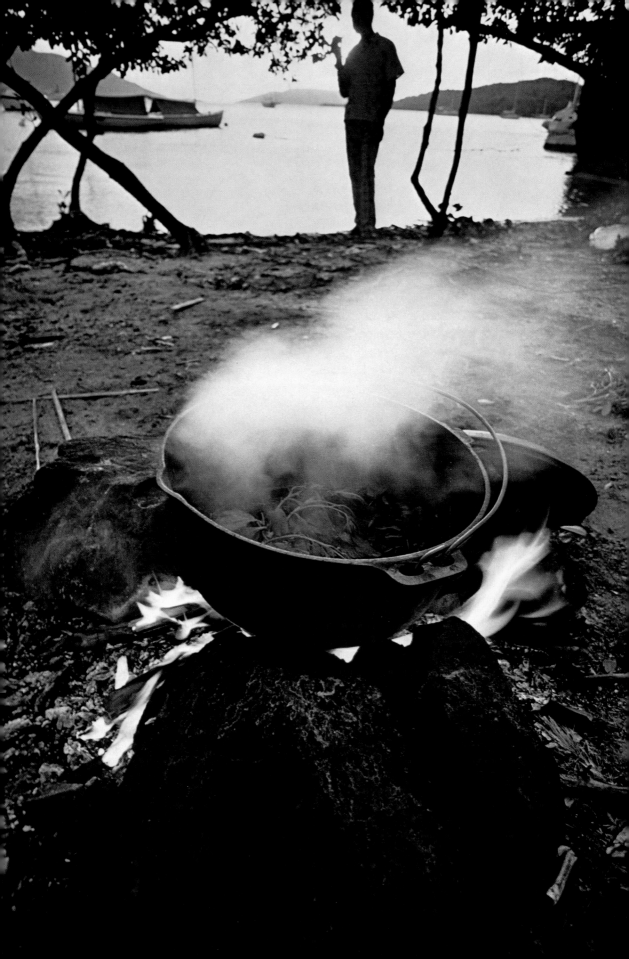

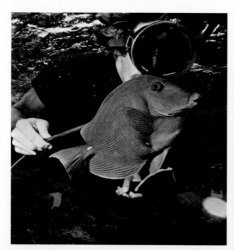

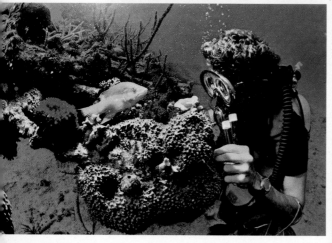

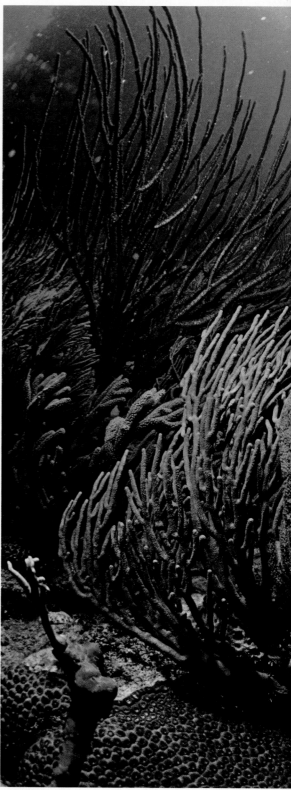

Exploring the untapped ocean realm, scientists in Virgin Gorda hope to discover new healing compounds—and clues to the mysterious origin of ciguatera. A diver descends into a colony of gorgonians—corals that may produce a potent antibiotic—to collect samples for laboratory study. Above, a marine pharmacognosist snips sponge tissue for bacterial research. At top, a diver carries a speared surgeonfish—a species that may harbor ciguatera toxins.

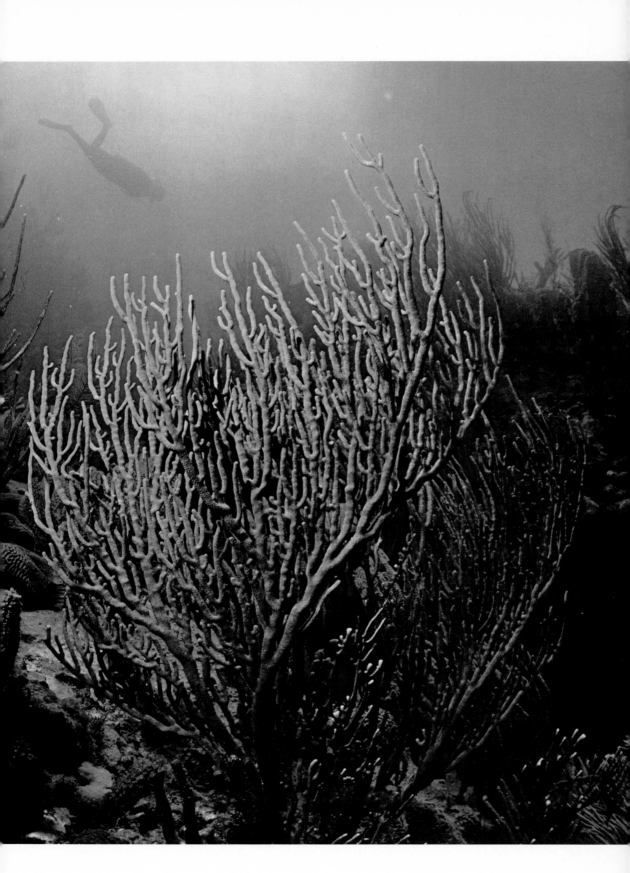

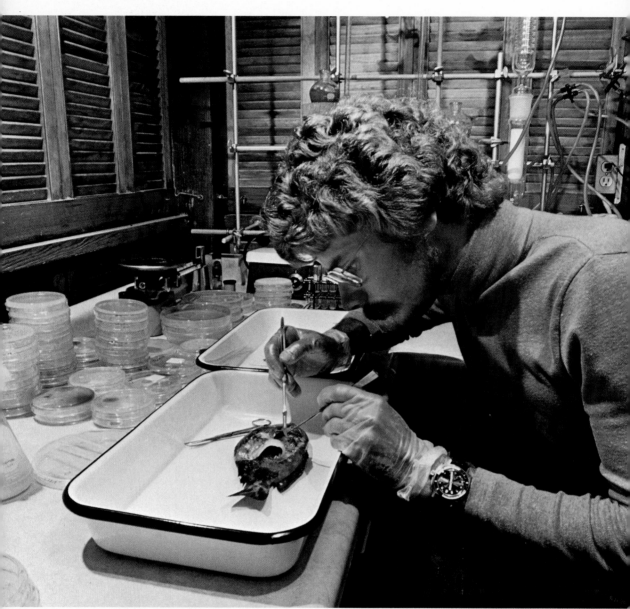

"The sea is potentially a rich source of drugs," says Ray Granade, a graduate student in pharmacognosy. Inside the Virgin Gorda laboratory, he dissects a surgeonfish to extract intestinal fluids. While testing these fluids for ciguatera toxins, he discovered "7RT"—a microorganism that may yield a new antibiotic. In a culture (right), a vertical smear of 7RT inhibits the growth of two of three lines of bacteria, demonstrating its strength.

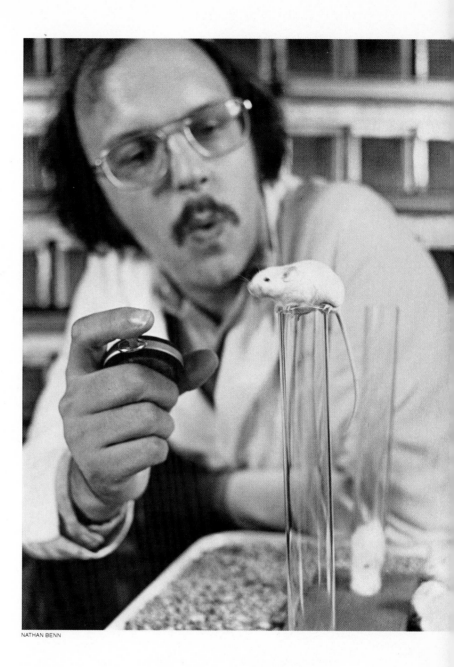

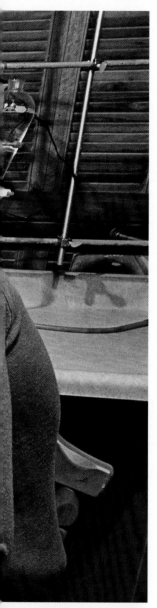

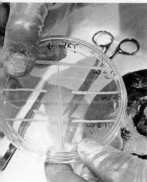

NATHAN BENN

Ciguatera research continues at the University of Mississippi, where Dr. Philip Wirth tests the performance of mice injected with toxins—one of many techniques used to determine the potency of marine specimens. With further study, scientists may harvest many new medicines from the ocean depths.

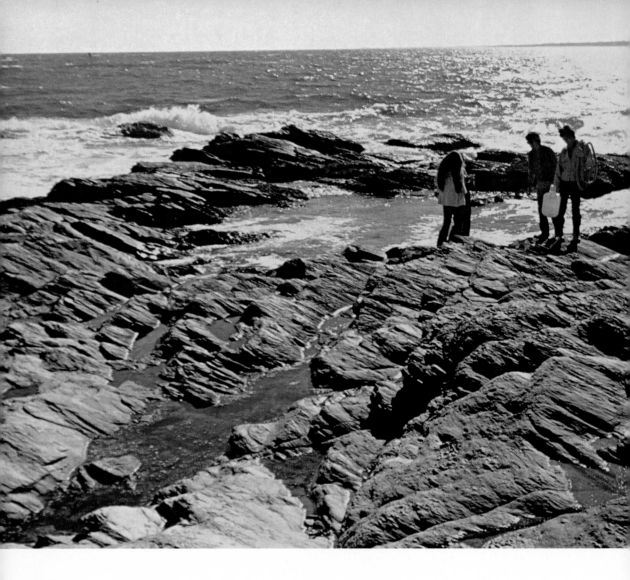

Working to solve the mystery of the red tide, Bill Fallon carries a jug of seawater for experiments at the University of Rhode Island. The deadly tide occurs when masses of tiny algae produce toxins and contaminate shellfish and other organisms that feed on them. Scientists hope soon to identify these toxins. In a refrigerated room at the university, Dr. Lawrence Buckley (right) shucks clams exposed to red tide, then points a scalpel at the dark gland where toxins accumulate. In another experiment (far right), Dr. Buckley isolates red algae compounds—studied for a possible cancer treatment.

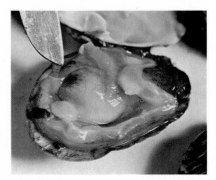

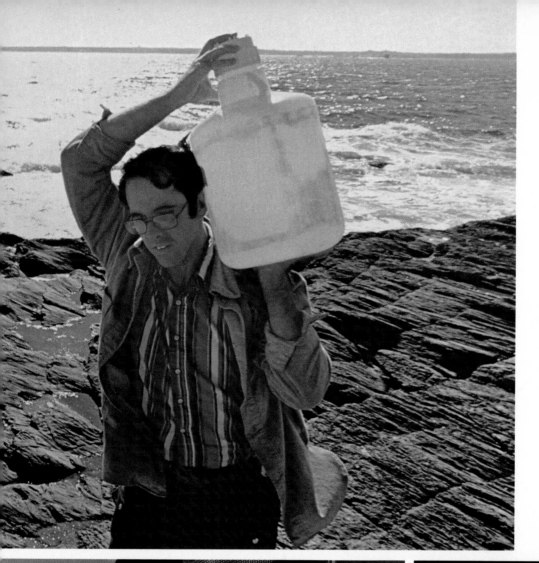

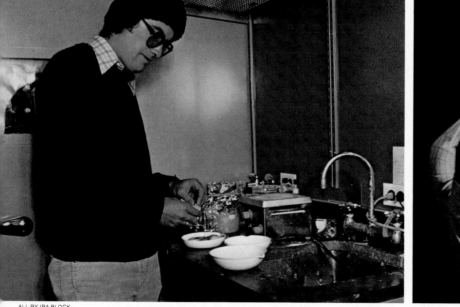

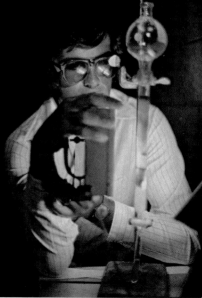

ALL BY IRA BLOCK

waded in. Now and then, they pulled out long, dripping seaweeds to be lugged back to the university in cardboard boxes. Once there, the plants would be dried and cleaned. Then would begin the complex laboratory procedures to isolate and purify any active substances they might contain.

One of the most exciting developments of the seaweed program, I learned, was the discovery that the species *Codium fragile* yields a substance that acts against certain types of leukemia cells. The University of Rhode Island's College of Pharmacy, the Medical School of Brown University, and the Roger Williams Hospital in Providence are working together to test the compound's effectiveness and safety.

In its other far-reaching project, the College of Pharmacy is researching the chemistry of the red tide, which, in different forms, affects many areas of the world.

The reddish color of the deadly tide comes from the blooming of myriad tiny organisms called dinoflagellates. This blooming produces toxins, which, when ingested by fish, often cause their death. At times, mass fish kills litter long stretches of the Atlantic and Pacific coasts. Red tide also brings serious illness—and occasionally respiratory paralysis—to people who eat shellfish that have absorbed the dinoflagellate poisons.

In fact, it was a massive red tide outbreak off the coast of New England in 1972 that prompted the university's investigations. The study began with the collection of toxic clams, Dr. Shimizu told me. He and his colleagues then cultured a supply of the dinoflagellates from which to extract the toxins.

"We're now beginning to reach a turning point in our work," he said. "The most important step is to identify the substances that cause the trouble. We've been rather successful in this, having isolated and purified six new toxins and established the chemical structure of two of them. Our next move will be to find a way to neutralize the toxins we've identified, and to develop either an antidote or a vaccine. Unfortunately, the only treatment so far available to a person suffering from the poison has been to provide a respirator to help the victim breathe.

"However, we're all hoping for a breakthrough. Other researchers also have identified toxins in the blooms, and still others are looking for the basic cause of the mass movement toward the shore, and for techniques to halt or dissipate it."

Marine biomedical science, as such, is only about 15 years old, having been held back by lack of proper equipment and the cost and hazards of exploring the oceans. Yet in that short time, enough research groups and institutions have taken up the subject to create a new world discipline.

Work in this field is now going on in countries from Japan to Sweden, from Mexico to Uganda to the Soviet Union. In the United States alone, more than a score of colleges of pharmacy and medical schools are engaged in undersea research. One of the leaders, strangely enough, is the landlocked University of Oklahoma.

Merely to list research groups and their projects hints at the scope of the inquiries. The University of Hawaii, for instance, is screening Pacific sponges that show activity against the highly infectious bacteria *Staphylococcus*. The University of Miami School of Medicine is looking into a group of spectacularly beautiful sea animals, the tunicates, which appear to be resistant to cancer, especially leukemia.

Several drug-manufacturing houses have set up underwater research branches, notably Switzerland's Hoffmann-La Roche, with its Roche Research Institute of Marine Pharmacology in Sydney, Australia. Also active in seagoing pharmacology are such prestigious organizations as the New York Aquarium, New York Zoological Society, and the Osborn Laboratories of Marine Sciences in Brooklyn; the National Science Foundation in Washington, D. C.; and the Scripps Institution of Oceanography in California.

Finally, as everyone's guide to the long-locked treasure chest of the deep, there is a definitive work entitled *Poisonous and Venomous Marine Animals of the World,* by Californian Bruce W. Halstead, a marine scholar, physician, diver, and former missionary. His three-volume encyclopedia covers 5,000 years of literature, biology, chemistry, and pharmacology on thousands of sea organisms.

Some medicinal products from the sea are already available. The following four were obtained, respectively, from a plant, a mammal, a fungus, and a fish. Sodium alginate, from kelp, can remove from the digestive system the dangerous nuclear-fission product Strontium 90. Spermaceti, a waxy substance from the head of the sperm whale, is used in ointments to treat skin ailments. Keflex, the trade name for a semi-synthetic antibiotic used against infections resistant to penicillin, was derived from a fungus found in sewage off the coast of Sardinia. And tetrodotoxin is a nerve-blocking substance that is one of the most powerful poisons known. Extracted from various parts of a fish called the puffer, this sea-born medication is prescribed only in tiny, supervised doses to relax muscle spasms and to relieve suffering in cases of terminal illness.

The example of the puffer is a reminder that the key to many biomedical chemicals from the sea—as is true of such land drugs as arrow poisons—lies in their toxicity. Strong poison indicates potent physiological and pharmacological effects. The ancient Sumerians made medications from pulverized skins of water snakes. Today, toxins from their venomous glands are under study as potential anesthetics.

On the milder side, salt water itself has been considered a healing agent for thousands of years. In his scholarly book, *The Healing Hand, Man and Wound in the Ancient World,* Guido Majno points out that Egyptians as early as 1550 B.C., applied salt in a poultice to "dry up the sore" of an infected chest wound.

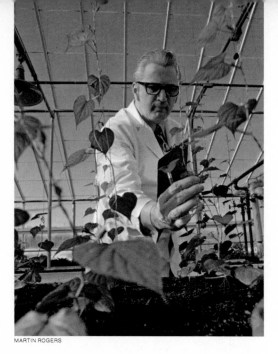

Yam vines frame Dr. Norman Farnsworth as he records their growth in a greenhouse at the University of Illinois in Chicago. Wild yams provide steroid-like substances that scientists can convert into cortisone and sex hormones. Now conducting a computerized study of plant drugs, Dr. Farnsworth says, "For every disease that afflicts mankind, there is a treatment or a cure occurring naturally on this earth."

In recent decades, a salt solution taken orally was found to be remarkably effective as a simple first-aid treatment for shock following severe burns or other bad injuries.

"The principle behind this treatment," explained Dr. Sanford Rosenthal, who led a 16-year study of the problem at the National Institutes of Health, "is the fact that blood plasma resembles seawater in its mineral composition. When an injury causes life-threatening shock by drawing large amounts of blood to the swollen trauma area, the saline solution replaces fluid and mineral content needed by the body to maintain its constituent balance."

Dr. Rosenthal's research on preventing fatal shock was launched by the U. S. Government during World War II to reduce deaths from battle wounds. For years, his experiments pushed uphill against the prevalent belief that blood plasma and proteins were the main lifesaving factors. But the salt solution won out, as is now clear, with many hospitals and doctors using it as standard procedure.

To compare ancient remedies with successful modern ones is not to say that scientists are picking daisies or fishing for drugs with hook and line. Still, the trend to look to the past is apparent.

In India, for instance, the World Health Organization is supporting a four-year study of traditional medicine in cooperation with the Indian Council of Medical Research. With herbal treatments carried on by practitioners of 3,000-year-old medicine, leaders of the program hope to find a cure for the painful and crippling disease of arthritis, which has so far defied the best efforts of science.

One of the reasons for increasing interest in traditional healing is the popularity and availability of medicinal plants in many nations that are short of cash and expertise. Consider the worldwide concern over regulating fertility to avoid overpopulation on the one hand, and to meet the desire of childless couples to become parents on the other.

Again, WHO is supporting research on folk medicine in countries that offer sources of plant chemicals with the hoped-for activity. In 1975 it pioneered the first major coordinated effort to develop fertility-regulating drugs from natural products, and it is now funding such projects in many nations. Professor Norman Farnsworth, a consultant for the Task Force on Indigenous Plants for Fertility Regulation of the Human Reproduction Unit of WHO, has assembled records of more than 3,000 species of plants. Some are simply from hearsay, but others have been checked by anthropologists, and a few validated by initial experiments with animals.

Dr. Farnsworth gathered this information and subsequently computerized it, using a method he developed and continues to use for the College of Pharmacy at the University of Illinois. In the eight years since the computer system was established, he also has compiled information on thousands of plants and other natural products with activity against diseases such as asthma, ulcers, diabetes, hepatitis, and sickle-cell anemia.

As part of his cooperation with WHO on the fertility-control project, Dr. Farnsworth presented 50 possible plant subjects from his computer collection for consideration by the Human Reproduction Unit at its meeting in Geneva in June 1977. Those chosen for preliminary study by the policy-making committee—which includes experts in such related fields as ethnobotany, pharmacognosy, biochemistry, toxicology, and reproductive pharmacology—are now beginning to be tested for their efficacy and suitability. Several plants in the original WHO program—*zoapatle,* for example, used for centuries by rural populations of Mexico—have been studied, and provide significant information that has reinforced the decision to enter this area of research.

"The plant kingdom has already supplied the starting material for the world's most widely used fertility-control drug—'The Pill,'" said Dr. Farnsworth. "This substance, diosgenin, is obtained from the Mexican yam of the *Dioscorea* genus, named for Dioscorides.

"The Pill, however, has highly controversial side effects," he added. "My hope is that we will soon find a plant that provides a harmless but effective contraceptive."

Birth—the renewal of life! Women who long for children have looked to plants as fertility aids in many times and places. One of the oldest herbs so sought was the mandrake, a member of the potato family, which grows abundantly in southern Europe and in the Bible lands.

In Genesis it is written that "Reuben went in the days of wheat harvest and found mandrakes. . . ." Rachel acquired them. "And she conceived, and bare a son."

To the ancients, mandrakes were objects of fear as well as of hope. It was believed that pulling up their roots, which resemble the human form, would bring unearthly shrieks from the plant and death to the violator.

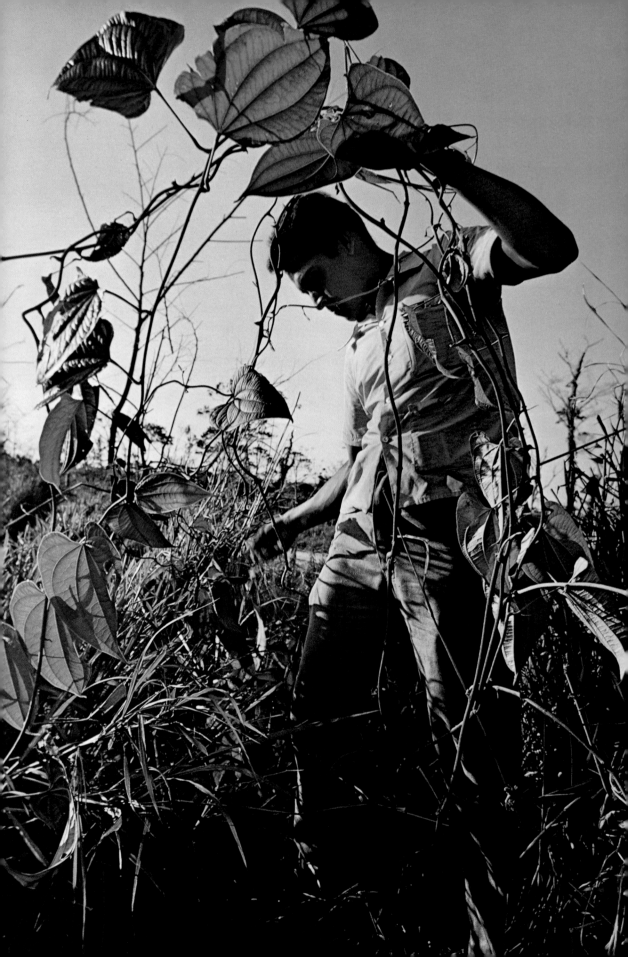

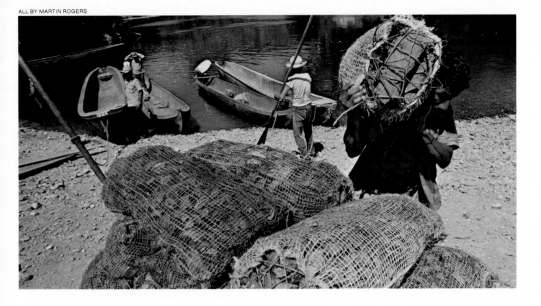

*Harvesting Mexican yams, a worker clears a vine to uncover the root—
source of the raw material for oral contraceptives. Above, laborers unload
bags of yam roots near a rural collection station in Mexico (below). As
many as 3,000 plants have served throughout history to regulate fertility;
scientists now reexamine many of these species for future use.*

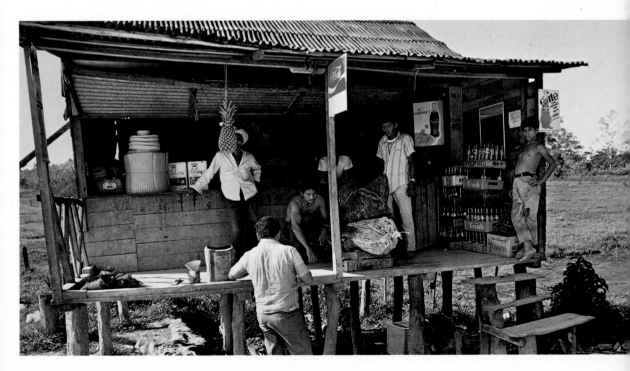

Therefore, an expendable dog was tied to the herb and made to drag it out of the ground. Recent analysis of mandrakes has revealed no active substance to support their reputation for aiding conception, says Dr. Farnsworth, although the root does, indeed, contain the alkaloids scopolamine and hyoscyamine.

Before scientists extracted nature's healing chemicals, midwives made scores of other plants into teas and salves to ease the pains and problems of childbearing before, during, and after delivery. Many of these plants have names familiar for other medicinal purposes: hollyhock, thyme, wormwood, burdock, slippery elm, smooth sumac, elder, mistletoe, and wahoo—to mention only a few.

Some were part of Indian birth lore in America's colonial days, passed on to pioneer families who bequeathed them to successive generations. A few yielded alkaloids that went into synthetic and semi-synthetic compounds of current obstetric practice. But the main source of such medications is ergot, a common fungus growth on grains, mostly rye.

Ergot derivations are valued because of their action in constricting blood vessels and causing muscular contractions that help control bleeding following birth. Though midwives of ancient and medieval times knew nothing of biomedical effects, they gained similar salutary results by giving crude preparations of the moldy grains to women in labor.

Ergot, however, is another product whose benefits must be weighed against the hazards of powerful blood-vessel constriction, which in severe cases can cause dry gangrene, with loss of hands or feet.

Mysterious plagues that struck rye-growing regions of Europe during the Middle Ages, and even in modern times, are now attributed to ergot poisoning. Usually due to eating mold-contaminated bread, this illness brought on terrifying hallucinations and illusions—symptomatic today of a "bad trip" caused by ingesting ergot's man-made offshoot, LSD.

Between the mysteries of birth and death, people find many ways to pursue the dream of perfect health and continued productivity. Juan Ponce de León was seeking the fabled Fountain of Youth when he landed on the wild shore of Florida and took possession in the name of Spain. Today the American way of life is still geared to youth, and the appearance of youth. Thus, many back-to-nature fans take vitamins and use drugs and cosmetics made from plants and other natural products of soil and sea.

Vitamins—whether taken voluntarily as food supplements or prescribed to correct deficiencies—have been widely used for only two decades or so, though their lack has caused diseases for centuries.

Scurvy, the occupational hazard of sailors deprived of fresh fruits and vegetables on long journeys, was the first of such diseases to be scientifically understood. In 1757 a British naval surgeon named James Lind proved that eating citrus fruits, which contain ample amounts of ascorbic acid, or vitamin C, would prevent or cure the disease. In 1795 the conservative British Admiralty finally decreed a daily ration of lemon or lime juice for its sailors—thus banishing scurvy from His Majesty's ships, and giving the nickname "limey" to British sailors.

Since then, 14 other vitamins have been recognized as essential: ten members of the vitamin B complex and the vitamins A, D, K, and E. Each plays a fractionally small but necessary role in preventing such diseases as beriberi, pellagra, and pernicious anemia. They also help counteract eye disorders, rickets, and hemorrhaging.

Controversies continue to rage over the merits of natural versus synthetic vitamins, and over taking massive doses to treat diseases. But all agree that their discovery has been a boon to ailing mankind.

To get a professional view of nutritive factors in the health and longevity of the elderly in America, I talked with Dr. Leroy E. Duncan, Jr., Special Projects Officer of the recently established National Institute on Aging. "So few nutritional studies of the elderly have been made," he said, "that we cannot exclude the possibility that they have significantly larger requirements for certain nutrients than do younger persons. Also, medical, social, or economic problems may result in inadequate amounts of vitamins and other nutrients in this group.

"The distinguished scientist and Nobel Laureate Dr. Linus Pauling has suggested that very large doses of vitamin C may be useful in improving the health of persons whose vitamin C intake already meets the usual standards. Several investigators also have suggested that vitamin E may retard aging. But evidence for both these views is uncertain, and it is not generally accepted by physicians. A number of natural agents, such as ginseng, also have been thought to retard the aging process, but, again, convincing evidence is lacking."

Some of nature's followers see clues to a long and productive life in the outdoor exercise and hard work of those sturdy centenarians who live in mountain pockets of the Soviet Caucasus, the Peruvian and Ecuadorean Andes, and the Himalayan land of Hunza.

Others cling to the familiar folk panaceas, or look to science to find good health and long life within our own bodies. Perhaps the answer lies in DNA, deoxyribonucleic acid, the genetic chemical in every living cell that helps determine our physical and mental characteristics.

During my year-long quest to learn of people, plants, and the healing arts, I met proponents of all these methods. At times their faces return to me in a kaleidoscope of images: Tibo Chavez gathering desert herbs; Robert Woodward delighting in the mysteries of molecules; Richard Evans Schultes discovering modern medicine in sacred potions of Amazonian Indians; Norman Farnsworth computerizing fertility drugs; Ray Granade diving for medicines. Each, in his own way, is seeking the "magic prescription" for good health. And each believes, as do I, that nature holds an increasingly bountiful trove of gifts up her green sleeve.

Worldwide search for natural drugs continues: At an Eli Lilly plant near Clinton, Indiana, scientists produce a powerful antibiotic that originated from a fungus found in sewage discharges off the coast of Sardinia. Arched pipes (below) pump air into fermentation tanks to grow antibiotic material. At right, a worker grips a high-pressure water hose used to clean one of the huge tanks. A flexible pneumatic tube (lower, right) sucks the antibiotic powder into containers for processing. The end product, Keflex, fights disease-causing bacteria, including those resistant to penicillin.

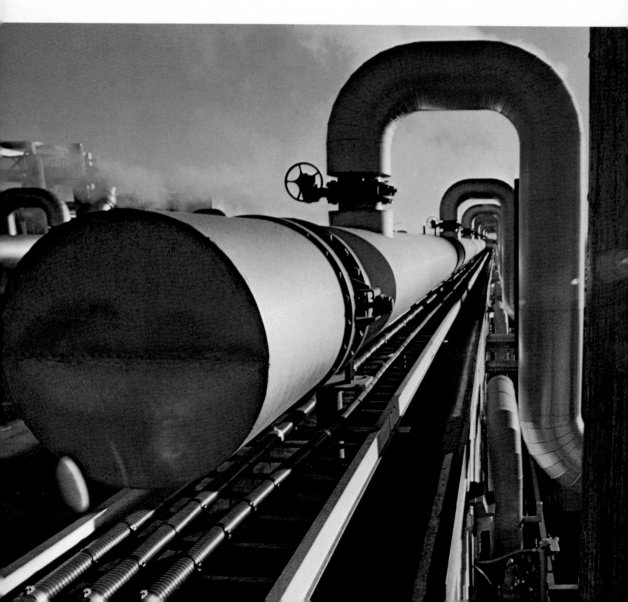

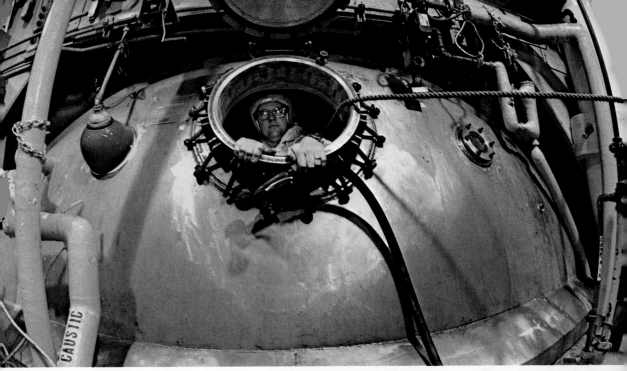

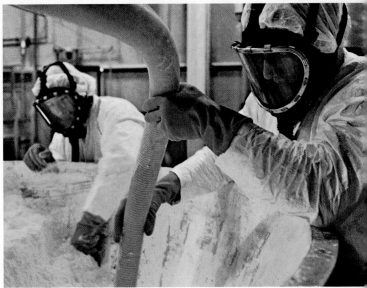

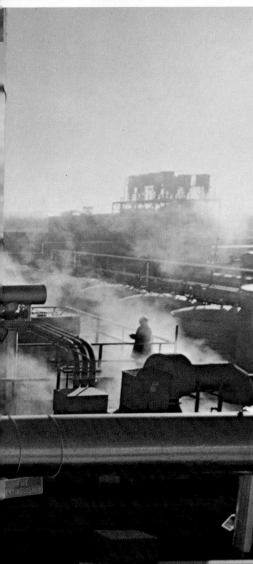

ALL BY NATHAN BENN

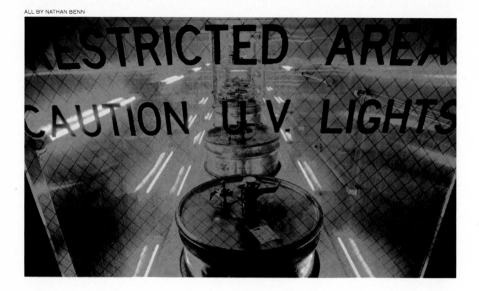

Drugs of the future depend on pioneering experiments today. Gazing into a vacuum chamber, Dr. Lee Ellis of Eli Lilly monitors the preparation of bacteria specimens for electron-microscope study. Above, ultraviolet light sterilizes drums of antibiotics before processing. Hundreds of glass tubes filled with solvents remove impurities from an antibiotic as a scientist extracts a sample for testing in a laboratory. Because of technological advances and an increasing awareness of the benefit of natural medicines, scientists today can unlock more and more of nature's healing secrets.

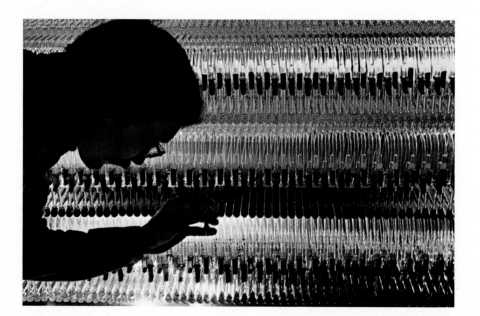

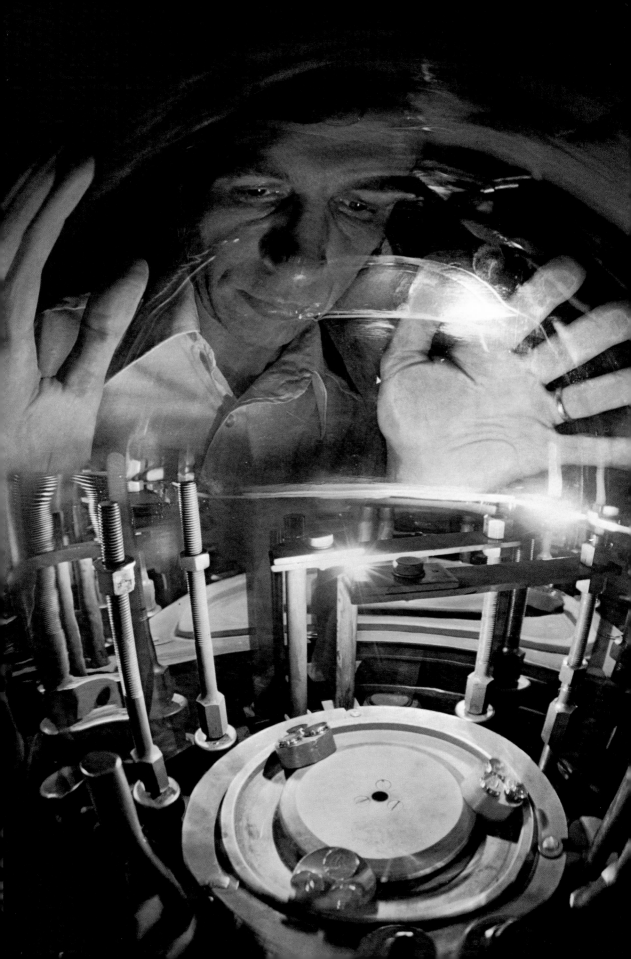

Acknowledgments

The Special Publications Division is grateful to the individuals, agencies, and organizations named or quoted in this book and to those cited here for their generous cooperation and help during its preparation: Dr. Ara Der Marderosian, Consultant; Dr. Thomas B. Hall, III; Dr. Norman R. Farnsworth; Dr. Miguel Civil; Prof. Dr. Med. F. H. Kemper; Dr. Paul McCullough; Earl Palmer; Dr. Guenter B. Risse; and Dr. Paul J. Scheuer. The American Pharmaceutical Association; Burroughs Wellcome Co.; Embassies of India, Kenya, Turkey, and Republic of China; Smithsonian Institution; U. S. Department of Agriculture, the National Arboretum; U. S. Department of Health, Education, and Welfare, Public Health Service: Center for Disease Control, National Institutes of Health, Public Health Service Hospitals; World Health Organization.

Additional Reading

The reader may wish to consult the *National Geographic Index* for related articles, and to refer to the following books: George A. Bender, *Great Moments in Medicine* and *Great Moments in Pharmacy;* Francesco Bianchini and Francesco Corbetta, *Health Plants of the World;* Daniel H. Efron, ed., *Ethnopharmacologic Search for Psychoactive Drugs;* Merritt Lyndon Fernald, *Gray's Manual of Botany;* Mildred Fielder, *Plant Medicine and Folklore;* Euell Gibbons, *Stalking the Healthful Herbs;* Mrs. M. Grieve, *A Modern Herbal;* Robert T. Gunther, *The Greek Herbal of Dioscorides;* B. Holmstedt and G. Liljestrand, eds., *Readings in Pharmacology;* John D. Keys, *Chinese Herbs;* Margaret B. Kreig, *Green Medicine;* Arnold and Connie Krochmal, *A Guide to the Medicinal Plants of the United States;* Geoffrey Marks and William K. Beatty, *The Medical Garden;* Cecilia C. Mettler, *History of Medicine;* Tony Swain, ed., *Plants in the Development of Modern Medicine;* Norman Taylor, *Plant Drugs That Changed the World;* Jürgen Thorwald, *Science and Secrets of Early Medicine;* Virgil J. Vogel, *American Indian Medicine;* Harold H. Webber and George D. Ruggieri, eds., *Food-Drugs From the Sea, 1974;* Michael A. Weiner, *Earth Medicine-Earth Foods* and *Man's Useful Plants;* R. W. Wren, ed., *Potter's New Cyclopaedia of Medicinal Herbs and Preparations.*

Composition for *Nature's Healing Arts: From Folk Medicine to Modern Drugs* by National Geographic's Photographic Services, Carl M. Shrader, Chief; Lawrence F. Ludwig, Assistant Chief. Printed and bound by Kingsport Press, Kingsport, Tenn. Color separations by Colorgraphics, Inc., Forestville, Md.; Graphic Color Plate, Inc., Stamford, Conn.; Graphic South, Charlotte, N.C.; Progressive Color Corp., Rockville, Md.; J. Wm. Reed Co., Alexandria, Va.

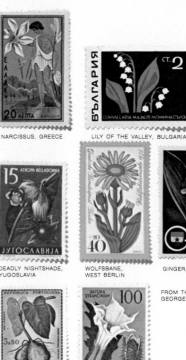

NARCISSUS, GREECE

LILY OF THE VALLEY, BULGARIA

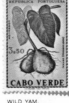

DEADLY NIGHTSHADE, YUGOSLAVIA

WOLFSBANE, WEST BERLIN

GINGER, GHANA

FROM THE COLLECTION OF GEORGE GRIFFENHAGEN

WILD YAM, CAPE VERDE

THORN APPLE, YUGOSLAVIA

With colorful postage stamps, nations salute medicinal plants.

Library of Congress CIP Data

Aikman, Lonnelle.   Nature's healing arts.
Bibliography: p.196;   Includes index.
1. Materia medica, Vegetable.   2. Folk medicine.   3. Pharmacognosy.
I. National Geographic Society, Washington, D. C., Special Publications Division.   II. Title.
RS164.A36   615'.32   76-56997   ISBN 0-87044-232-5

Scientific Names of Important Plants and Animals that Provide Medicinal Remedies

Plants

Alfalfa, *Medicago sativa*
Aloe, *Aloe vera*
Asafetida, *Ferula foetida*
Autumn crocus, *Colchicum autumnale*
Bloodroot, *Sanguinaria canadensis*
Boneset, *Eupatorium perfoliatum*
Burdock, *Arctium lappa*
Buttonwood, *Conocarpus erecta*
Calamus, *Acorus calamus*
Catnip, *Nepeta cataria*
Chamomile, *Anthemis nobilis*
Chaulmoogra tree, *Taraktogenus Kurzii*
Cherry, wild, *Prunus serotina*
Cinnamon, *Cinnamomum zeylanicum*
Coca bush, *Erythroxylum coca*
Comfrey, *Symphytum officinale*
Dandelion, *Taraxacum officinale*
Datura, African, *Datura metel*
Datura, tree, *Datura sanguinea*
Deadly nightshade (Belladonna), *Atropa belladonna*
Dittany, *Cunila mariana*
Dock, *Rumex crispus*
Elder, *Sambucus nigra*
Ephedra, *Ephedra sinica*

Foxglove, *Digitalis purpurea*
Ginger, *Zingiber officinale*
Ginseng, American, *Panax quinquefolium*
Ginseng, red, *Panax ginseng*
Golden seal, *Hydrastis canadensis*
Henbane, *Hyoscyamus niger*
Hollyhock, *Althaea rosea*
Horehound, *Marrubium vulgare*
Horsemint, *Monarda punctata*
Horsetail reed, *Equisetum arvense*
Ipecac, *Cephaelis ipecacuanha*
Jamaica dogwood, *Piscidia erythrina*
Jimsonweed, *Datura stramonium*
Lamb's-quarters, *Trillium erectum*
Licorice, *Glycyrrhiza glabra*
Life everlasting, *Antennaria dioica*
Lizard's-tail herb, *Saururus cernuus*
Madagascar periwinkle,
    Catharanthus roseus (Vinca rosea)
Mandrake, *Atropa mandragora*
Marijuana, *Cannabis sativa*
Mayapple, *Podophyllum peltatum*
Milk vetch, *Astragalus mongolicus*
Mistletoe, *Viscum album*
Morning glory, *Rivea corymbosa*
Mullein, *Verbascum thapsus*

Mushroom, *Psilocybe mexicana*
Neem tree, *Azadirachta indica*
Osha, *Ligusticum porteri*
Pennyroyal, *Mentha pulegium*
Peppermint, *Mentha piperita*
Peyote, *Lophophora williamsii*
Pleurisy root, *Asclepias tuberosa*
Pokeroot, *Phytolacca americana*
Pomegranate, *Punica granatum*
Poppy, *Papaver somniferum*
Purslane, *Portulaca oleracea*
Sage, *Salvia officinalis*
Sarsaparilla, *Smilax glauca*
Sassafras, *Sassafras albidum*
Securinega, *Securinega suffruticosa*
Showy alpinia, *Alpinia speciosa*
Slippery elm, *Ulmus fulva*
Smooth sumac, *Rhus glabra*
Snakeroot, Virginia, *Aristolochia serpentaria*
Spearmint, *Mentha spicata*
Squill, *Urginea maritima*
Strychnine, *Strychnos nux-vomica*
Sweet flag, *Acorus calamus*
Tasselflower, *Emilia sonchifolia*
Thorn apple, *Datura stramonium*
Turpentine weed, *Aletris farinosa*

Violet, *Viola odorata*
Wahoo, *Euonymus atropurpurea*
Water lily, *Nymphaea spp.*
Wild mint, *Mentha sativa*
Willow, *Salix alba*
Wormseed, *Chenopodium ambrosioides*
Wormwood, *Artemisia absinthium*
Yam, Mexican, *Dioscorea composita*
Yam, wild, *Dioscorea distachya*
Yarrow, *Achillea millefolium*
Yellowroot, *Berberis vulgaris*
Yucca, *Agave spp.*
Zoapatle, *Montanoa tomentosa*

Animals

Caribbean sponge, *Haliclona spp.*
Clam, *Mya arenaria*
Goatfish, *Upeneus arge*
Puffer, *Tetraodon spp.*
Queen conch, *Strombus gigas*
Red tide, *Gonyaulax tamarensis*
Sea cucumber, *Actinopyga agassizi*
Sea wasp, *Chiropsalmus quadrumanus*
Surgeonfish, *Acanthurus spp.*
Toad, *Bufo vulgaris*

Index

Boldface indicates illustrations;
Italic refers to picture legends (captions)

198

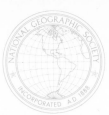

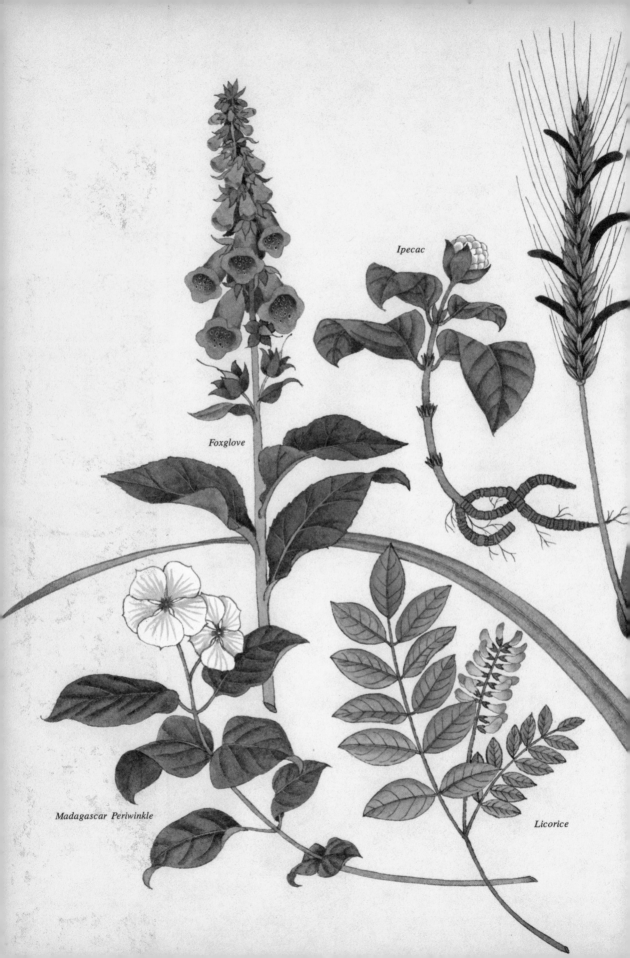

Foxglove

Ipecac

Madagascar Periwinkle

Licorice